The A to Z of Surface Anatomy

Introduction

This book describes the structures which lie beneath the skin. It involves a recognition of the surface markings of most skeletal muscles, hence it ties in well with *the A to Z of Skeletal Muscles*, and of course *the A to Z of the Hair, Nails and Skin*. All ***the A to Zs*** are cross-referenced and together are forming a comprehensive set of reference books covering the structural elements of the human body. Recently pathology as well as anatomy has been tackled by ***the A to Zs*** with *the A to Z of Bone & Joint Failure* the first book to cover the breakdown of the body's structures in this manner, expanding upon the knowledge of *the A to Z of Bones, Joints, Ligaments and the Back*. It is planned to expand and include a companion ***A to Z of the failure of …*** for the other A to Zs.

If there is a structure / subject you want to see in the A to Zs let us know. All feedback is appreciated.

anatomy.update@gmail.com

The A to Zs and additional material may be viewed on the following sites **http://www.aspenpharma.com.au/atlas/student.htm** **www.amandasatoz.com**

Acknowledgement

Thank you Aspenpharmacare Australia for your support and assistance in this valuable project, particularly Greg Lan, and Rob Koster. Thank you to all those who have helped when I have been rushed to finish and have made time for this project. Thank you everyone who has provided feedback it is always appreciated. Thank you, Richard, Peter, Robbie, Jody, Quentin and all the others.

Dedication

To those who read and use these books and find them helpful

How to use this book

The structure of the A to Zs grows and develops with each new book while the principle of listing structures in an alphabetical is maintained. Basic anatomical concepts are placed in the beginning of this book; then measurements and proportions of the body. The role of the Common Terms section is enlarged, illustrated and colour coded.

In this book the images are alphabetical whether they can be seen or not – i.e. the heart cannot be seen but its projection are indicated on the chest – but the tendons of the wrist can be visualized. All entries are cross referenced in the usual manner i.e. ***see*** for ***go to*** and ***also see*** for ***additional images listed under that heading***.

The back cover has been modified in all the new editions of the A to Zs to include an additional **fold over** which serves as a means of identifying the book on the shelf (i.e. the fold over has the title down the "spine"). Hence the spiral binding is preserved, but the book can easily be identified if this **fold over** is placed outward in the bookshelf.

The fold over may also be used as a **fold in / bookmark** and it is designed to lay flat if folded over onto the back cover.

Thank you

A.L. Neill
BSc MSc MBBS PhD FACBS
medicalamanda@gmail
ISBN 978-1-921930-17-1

Table of contents

Index of Surface Anatomy

Abbreviations

A = atrium, (pl atria) / actions / movements of a joint
a = artery
abdo = abdomen / abdominal
ACF = anterior cranial fossa
adj. = adjective
AIIS = anterior inferior iliac spine
aka = also known as
alt. = alternative
AM = arachnoid mater
ANS = autonomic nervous system
ant = anterior
art. = artery
AS = Alternative Spelling, generally referring to the diff. b/n British & American spelling
ASIS = anterior superior iliac spine
assoc. = associated with
AV = atrioventricular
B = blood
BBB = blood brain barrier
bc = because
BF = blood flow
BM = basement membrane
b/n = between
BP = brachial plexus
bpm = beats per minute
br = branch (of a vessel)
BS = blood supply / blood stream
BV = blood vessel(s)
cap. = capillary
c.f. = compared to
C = carpal
C = cervical
CC = costal border
CC = costal cartilage
CH = cerebral hemispheres
cm = cell membrane
CNS = central nervous system
collat. = collateral
CP = cervical plexus
Cr = cranial
CSF = Cerebrospinal fluid
CT = connective tissue
CVA = cerebrovascular accident = stroke
defn = definition
diff. = difference(s)
dist. = distal
DM = dura mater
DVT = deep vein thrombosis
EAM = external auditory meatus
e.g. = example
EC = extracellular (outside the cell)
ECG = electrocardiogram
ED = extensor digitorum
ER = Extensor Retinaculum
FDP = Flexor digitorum porofundus
FDS = Flexor digitorum superficialis
FPB = Flexor pollicus brevis
FPL = Flexor pollicus longus
FR = Flexor Retinaculum
Gk. = Greek
H = hormone(s)
H = hypochondrium
HB = heart beat
HF = heart failure
HR = heart rate
HS = heart sounds
IC = intercostal
IC = intercarpal
ICS = intercostal space
IP = interphalangeal
Ix = investigation
IVC = inferior vena cava
jt(s) = joints = articulations
L = left
L = lumbar
LA = Left Atrium
lat. = lateral
LH = left hypochondrium
LL = lower limb
LIF = left iliac fossa
lig = ligament
Lt. = Latin
m = muscle
MC = metacarpal
MCF = middle cranial fossa

MCL = mid clavicular line
MCP = metacarpophalangeal
med. = medial
MI = myocardial infarction
MIP = midinguinal point
MT = metatarsal
N = nerve
NAD = normal (size, shape)
NAD = no abnormality detected
NR = nerve root
NS = nervous system/nerve supply
NT = nervous tissue
nv = neurovascular bundle
P = pressure
PAD = peripheral artery disease
PaNS = parasympathetic nervous system
Ph = phalanges
PIIS = posterior inferior iliac spine
pl. = plural
PM = pia mater
PN = peripheral nerve
post. = posterior
proc. = process
prox. = proximal
PS = pubic symphysis
PSIS = posterior superior iliac spine
R = right
RA = right atrium
RH = right hypochondrium
RIF = Right Iliac Fossa
S = sacral
S1 = first heart sound
S2 = second heart sound
SA = sinoatrial
SCM = sternocleidomastoid muscle
sing. = singular
SC = spinal cord
SN = spinal nerve
SP = spinal process
SR = sarcoplasmic reticulum
subcut. = subcutaneous
supf = superficial
SVC = superior vena cava
SyNS = sympathetic nervous system
T = thoracic
TMJ = temporomandibular joint
UL = upper limb, arm
V = vertebra
V = ventricle
VC = vertebral column
WM = white matter
w/n = within
w/o = without
wrt = with respect to
& = and
∩ = intersection with

Common Terms used in Surface Anatomy

Ablation the removal of part of the body, generally a bony part, most commonly the teeth

Acromegaly a continuation of growth of the ends of cartilage covered bone (after fusion of the long bones) hence a gross change in the features (most noticeable in the jaw and digits) without growth in height, due mainly to the over activity of the pituitary gland

Ala a wing, hence a wing-like process as in the Ethmoid bone *pl. - alae. Alveolus* Air filled bone - tooth socket adj - alveolar (as in air filled bone in the maxilla)

Aneurysm a localized dilatation of an artery or heart chamber caused by disease or weakening of the muscle in the wall – tunica media.

Angina/Angina Pectoris chest pain or discomfort due to lack of oxygen - anoxia or ischemia in the muscle tissue (myocardium) generally bc of coronary artery disease. Angina is a symptom of a condition called myocardial ischemia; may also manifest as : aching, burning, discomfort, heaviness, numbness, pressure, tightness, *and/or* tingling in the chest, back, neck, throat, jaw or arms.

Angiography an X-ray that uses dye injected into arteries so that coronary artery anatomy can be studied wrt disease diagnosis.

Ankle bend = angle usually referring to the bend just above the foot, hence the ankle is the joint b/n the foot and the lower leg

Aorta the largest artery in the body and the primary BV leading from the heart to the body.

Aortic Valve the valve that regulates BF from the heart to the aorta.

Aperture an opening or space between bones or within a bone.

Apex (of the Heart) the inferior aspect or bottom of the heart 5th ICS, L MCL, where the HB is the strongest

Appendicular refers to the appendices of the axial i.e. in the skeleton, the limbs upper and lower which hang from the axial skeleton, this also includes the pectoral and pelvic girdles (not the Sacrum) adj. appendicular

Areola small, open spaces as in the areolar part of the Maxilla may lead or develop into sinuses. *pl. areolae*

Artery a BV that carries blood away from the heart.

Arth- to do with joints hence…

Articulation joint, description of the bone surfaces joining w/o the supporting structures = point of contact b/n 2 opposing bones hence the articulation of Humerus and Scapula is the articulation of the shoulder joint.

Auditory exostosis a bony growth on the walls of the EAM

Atrium	Lt antrum = waiting room – top chambers R & L of the heart - 1/3 of the volume of the Ventricle or lower chamber. Blood flows from the atria to the Ventricles.
Avulsion	forceable tearing away of a structure or part of a structure as in an avulsed fracture where a fragment bone is torn away from the main bone
Axis	of the body - is the central part - the line through the head & spine, the axial skeleton as opposed to the appendicular
Base - "of the Heart"	top of the heart located in the 4th ICS
Basilar	relating to the base or bottom of structures
Basiocranium	bones of the base of the skull
Boss	a smooth round broad eminence - mainly in the frontal bone female > male
Bregma	refers to a junction of more than 2 bones in a joint as in the Bregma of the skull, junction between the coronal and sagittal sutures which in the infant is not closed and can be felt pulsating – site of the anterior fontanelle.
Buccal	pertaining to the cheek
Calotte	consists of the Calvaria from which the base has been removed.
Calvaria	refers to the Cranium without the facial bones attached.
Canal	tunnel / extended foramen as in the carotid canal at the base of the skull *adj canular* (canicular - small canal)
Caput / Kaput	the head or of a head, *adj.- capitate* = having a head (c.f. decapitate)
Carotid	to put to sleep; compression of the common or internal carotid artery causes coma.
Carpo	wrist
Catheter	a thin, flexible tube
Cavity	an open area or sinus within a bone or formed by two or more bones *(adj. cavernous)*, may be used interchangeably with fossa. Cavity tends to be more enclosed fossa a shallower bowl like space (Orbital fossa-Orbital cavity).
Cavum	a cave.
Cephalic	pertaining to the head
Cervico	pertaining to the neck
Concha	a shell shaped bone as in the ear or nose *(pl. conchae adj. chonchoid)* old term for this turbinate.
Condyle	a rounded enlargement or process possessing an articulating surface.
Cornu	a horn (as in the Hyoid)

Corona a crown. *adj.- coronary,* coronoid or coronal; hence a coronal plane is parallel to the main arch of a crown which passes from ear to ear (c.f. coronal suture).

Costo/Costa pertaining to the ribs

Conductivity the ability to conduct an impulse to another region or another cell

Congenital existing at birth.

Congestive heart failure blood volume coming in is more than that pumped out - leading to fluid backup - backup from the LV results in fluid overload in the lungs - in the RV results in venous fluid retention and then swelling of dependant parts

Coronary Arteries two arteries arising from the aorta that arch down over the top of the heart and branch out in additional arteries that provide B to the heart muscle – the main 4 being L main coronary artery, Circumflex coronary artery, L ant descending coronary artery, and R coronary artery. They join to form rings around the heart b/n the A & Vs and b/n the 2 Vs. These are the most commonly blocked arteries of the heart.

Cranium comprises all of the bones of the skull except for the Mandible.

Crest prominent sharp thin ridge of bone formed by the attachment of muscles particularly powerful ones eg Temporalis/Sagittal crest

Cuneate /Cuneus a wedge / wedge-shaped

Dens a tooth hence dentine and dental relating to teeth, denticulate having tooth-like projections *adj dentate See odontoid*

Depression a concavity on a surface

Diaphysis The shaft or body of a long bone. In the young this is the region between the growth plates & is composed of compact bone. *pl.= diaphyses adj.= diaphyseal*

Diploë the cancellous bone between the inner and outer tables of the skull, *adj.- diploic.*

Echocardiogram a study using high-frequency sound waves to picture or visualize the heart chambers, the thickness of the muscle wall, the heart valves and major BVs located near the heart. This is a non-invasive procedure.

Edentulous without teeth

Elbow any angular bend often in the arm, usually referring to the joint between the arm and the forearm

Eminence a smooth projection or elevation on a bone as in iliopubic eminence.

Endocranium refers to the interior of the "braincase" divided into the 3 major fossae anterior (for the Frontal lobes) middle (containing Temporal lobes) & posterior (for the containment of the Cerebellum).

Epiphysis the end of a long bone beyond the growth plate or epiphyseal plate. Generally develops as a secondary ossification centre. There are 2 epiphyses to each long bone. Of a long bone the shafts are generally compact bone and the ends=epiphyses are trabecular bone *adj.= epiphyseal*

External Auditory Meatus ear hole

Exostosis a bony outgrowth from a bony surface, often due to irritation (as in swimmer's ear) and may involve ossification of surrounding tissues such as muscles or ligaments.

Facet a face, a small bony surface (occlusal facet on the chewing surfaces of the teeth) seen in planar joints.

Falciform relating to shapes that are in a sickle shape so falciform ligaments curve around and end in a sharp point

Fissure a narrow slit or gap from cleft.

Fontanelle a fountain, associated with the palpable pulsation of the brain as in the anterior fontanelle of an infant. these soft spots on the skull are cartilagenous connective tissue coverings "joints" which allow for skull cranial expansion and then become the mould for the bone development and shape joining long the sutural lines, later becoming the Bregma.

Foramen a natural hole in a bone usually for the transmission of blood vessels and/or nerves. *(pl. foramina).*

Fornix an arch

Fossa a pit, depression, or concavity, on a bone, or formed from several bones as in temporomandibular fossa. Shallower and more like a "bowl" than a cavity

Fovea a small pit (usually smaller than a fossa)- as in the fovea of the occlusal surface of the molar tooth.

Genu / genio referring to the knee

Groove long pit or furrow

Hallux the big toe = the first toe

Hamus a hook hence the term used for bones which "hook around other bones or where other structures are able to attach by hooking - hamulus = a small hook.

Hyoid U-shaped

Incisura a notch.

Inter between

Intra within

Introitus an orifice or point of entry to a cavity or space.

Joint = Articulation supporting structures

Lacerum something lacerated, mangled or torn e.g. foramen lacerum small sharp hole at the base of the skull - often ripping tissue in trauma.

Lacrimal related to tears and tear drops. *(noun lacrima)*

Lambda Greek letter a capital 'L' - written as an inverted\ V.(adj. lambdoid) - used to name the point of connection b/n 3 skull bones Occipital and L & R Temporal bones.

Lamina a plate as in the lamina of the Vertebra a plate of bone connecting the vertical and transverse spines *(pl. laminae)*

Ligament a band of tissue which connects bones (articular ligaments) or viscera - organs (visceral ligaments).

Linea a line as in the Nuchal lines of the Occitipum

Lingual pertaining to the tongue

Locus a place (c.f. location, locate, dislocate).

Lymphatic a vessel which carries fluid to the heart

Magnum large *pl magna*

Malleus hammer (as in the ear ossicle)

Mandible from the verb to chew, hence, the movable lower jaw; *adj.- mandibular.*

Mastoid breast or teat shape - mastoid process of the Temporal bone.

Maxilla the jaw-bone; now used only for the upper jaw; *adj.- maxillary.*

Meatus a short passage; *adj.- meatal* as in external acoustic meatus connecting the outer ear with the middle ear.

Mediastinum the region in the thorax b/n the lungs, ant. boundary- the sternum post. the VC, includes the heart, roots of the great vessels, oesophagus and trachea.

Meniscus Gk. crescent as in the crescent shaped cartlages on the top of the Tibia

Mental relating to the chin (mentum = chin not mens = mind).

Meta an extension of: cf. metacarpal = extension of the wrist

Metaphysis the slightly expanded end of the shaft of a bone.

Microvasculature the network of small BVs arterioles ⇨capillaries ⇨venules in a tissue

Minimally Invasive Heart Surgery a variety of approaches using smaller incisions to reduce the trauma of surgery and potentially speed recovery.

Mitral Valve the valve that controls the BF b/n the LA & LV in the heart.

Murmur a specific sound emanating from the chest in addition to the normal HS.

Myocardial Infarct also called "heart attack"; the sudden interruption or insufficiency of the supply of B to the heart, typically resulting from occlusion or obstruction of a coronary artery and often characterized by severe chest pain

Myocardial infarction death of myocardial tissue due to anoxia .

Neurocranium	the neurocranium refers only to the braincase of the skull.
Non-invasive procedure	a procedure that can be done outside of the body, such as an X-ray or ECG.
Notch	an indentation in the margin of a structure.
Nucha	the nape or back of the neck *adj.- nuchal.*
Occiput	the prominent convexity of the back of the head Occipitum = Occipital bone *adj. occipital*
Occulus	an eye
Odontoid	relating to teeth, toothlike see Dens
Orbit	a circle; the name given to the bony socket in which the eyeball rotates; *adj - orbital.*
Orifice	an opening.
Os	a bone or pertaining to bones *adj osseus*
Ossification	the process of turning something into bone, i.e. from one tissue to another as in cartilagneous ossification from cartilage into bone
Ostium	a door, an opening, an orifice.
Otic	pertaining to the ear
Ovale	oval shaped
Palate	a roof *adj.- palatal or platatine.*
Palpitation	irregular HB that can be felt by a person.
Parietal	pertaining to the outer wall of a cavity from paries, a wall.
Parotid	pertaining to a region beside or near the ear
Pars	a part of
Pecten	a comb.
Perikymata	transverse ridges and the grooves on the surfaces of teeth
Periosteum	layer of fascial tissue connective tissue on the outside of compact bone not present on articular (joint) surfaces see endostium
Petrous	pertaining to a rock / rocky / stoney *adj. petrosal*
Phalanx	pertaining to flanks of soldiers - phalanges a row of soldiers used for a row of fingers or toes
Pollex	thumb
Process	a general term describing any marked projection or prominence as in the mandibular process.
Prominens	a projection
Pseudoarthrosis	false or new joint due to the nonhealing of a fracture
Pterion	a wing; the region where the tip of the greater wing of the sphenoid meets or is close to the parietal, separating the frontal from the squamous region of the temporal bone.
Pubis	hairy, that part of the hip bone with hair over the surface *adj pubic pl pubes*

Pulmonary Valve the heart valve located b/n the RV and the pulmonary artery that controls BF to the lungs.

Ramus branch as in the superior pubic ramus the superior or higher branch of the pubic bone

Recess a secluded area or pocket; a small cavity set apart from a main cavity.

Rectus straight - erect

Ridge elevated bony growth often roughened.

Rotundum Round

Sagittal an arrow, the sagittal suture is notched posteriorly, making it look like an arrow by the lambdoid sutures.

Sesamoid grainlike

Sigmoid S-shaped, from the letter Sigma which is S in Greek.

Sinus a space usually within a bone lined with mucous membrane, such as the frontal and maxillary sinuses in the head, (also, a modified BV usually vein with an enlarged lumen for blood storage and containing no or little muscle in its wall). Sinuses may contain air, venous or arterial blood, lymph or serous fluid depending upon location and health of the subject *adj.- sinusoid.*

Skull refers to all of the bones that comprise the head.

Spheno a wedge i.e. the Sphenoid is the bone which wedges in the base of the skull between the unpaired frontal and occipital bones *adj. - sphenoid.*

Spine a thorn *adj. - spinous* descriptive of a sharp, slender process/protrusion.

Splanchocranium the splanchocranium refers to the facial bones of the skull.

Sulcus long wide groove often due to a BV indentation

Sustenaculum a supportive structure as in the sustenaculum tali = a structure which supports the Talus in the foot

Suture The saw-like edge of a cranial bone that serves as joint between bones of the skull.

Stylos an instrument for writing hence *adj. - styloid* a pencil-like structure.

Symphysis a cartilagenous joint or a growth with bone-cartilage-bone

Syn together in the close proximity of or fusion of 2 structures

Syndesmosis tight inflexible joints b/n 2 bones little to no movement many axial joints

Synostosis fusion of any joints

Synovial joint any moveable joint with synovial fluid b/n the 2 opposing bones - most moving joints are synovial

Talus ankle (Gk. bend)

Tarsus	pertaining to any bones joining the foot with the leg *adj. - tarsal* (Gk wickerwork referring to the basketlike structure of the os tarsus with the ligaments)
Temporal	refers to time and the fact that grey hair (marking the passage of time) often appears first at the site of the temporal bone.
Tendon	a tie or cord of collagen fibres connecting muscle with bone (as opposed to articular ligaments which connect bone with bone)
Tentorium	a tent.
Trabecula	a “little” beam i.e. supporting structure or strut *pl. trabeculae*
Tricuspid Valve	the heart valve that controls the BF from the RA into the RV.
Trochanter	pertaining to a small wheel or disc, in the Femur it is a large disc shaped tuberosity
Trochlea	a pulley that part of the bone or ligamantous attachment that pulls the bone in another direction as in the elbow or the ankle
Tubercle	a small process or bump, an eminence..
Tuberculum	a very small prominence, process or bump.
Tuberosity	a large rounded process or eminence, a swelling or large rough prominence often associated with a tendon or ligament attachment.
Turbinate	a child’s spinning top, hence shaped like a top; an old term for the nasal conchae.
Tympanum	a drum *pl. tympani*
Uncus	a hook *adj. - uncinate.*
Vagal maneuver	stimulation of the vagal N to decrease HR and BP may cause fainting
Vagina	A sheath; hence, invagination is the acquisition of a sheath by pushing inwards into a structure, and evagination is similar but produced by pushing outwards *adj. - vaginal.*
Valve	there are 4 heart valves: mitral, aortic, pulmonary and tricuspid, that act as one-way "doors" between the chambers of the heart.
Vein	a BV which carries B to the heart
Ventricles	lower heart 2 chambres – 3X the volume of the atria
Wormian bone	extrasutural bone in the skull
Zygoma	a yoke , hence, the bone joining the maxillary, frontal, temporal & sphenoid bones *adj zygomatic.*

Anatomical Planes and Relations

This is the anatomical position.

A = Anterior Aspect from the front = or / Posterior Aspect from the back. Used interchangeably with ventral and dorsal respectively

B = Lateral Aspect from either side

C = Transverse / Horizontal plane

D = Midsagittal plane = Median plane; trunk moving away from this plane = lateral flexion or lateral movement.-
plane medial movement; limbs moving away from this direction = abduction; limbs moving closer to this plane = adduction

E = Coronal plane

F = Median

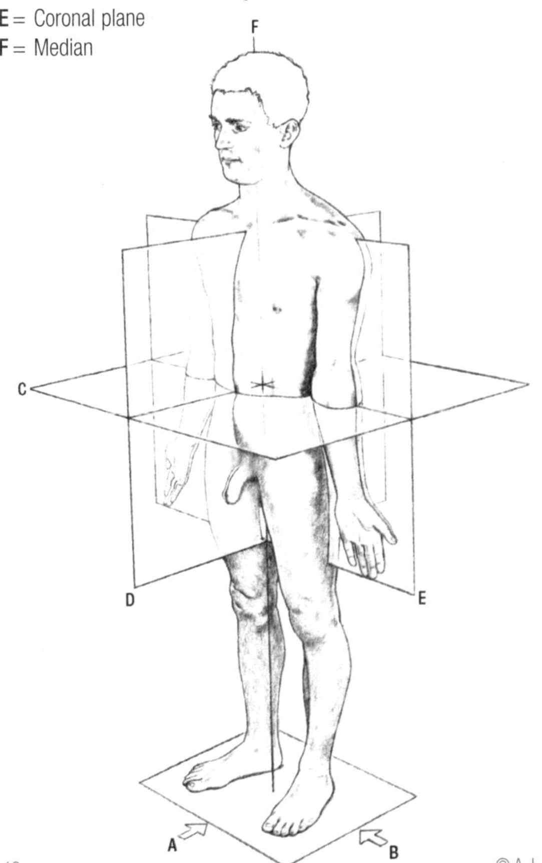

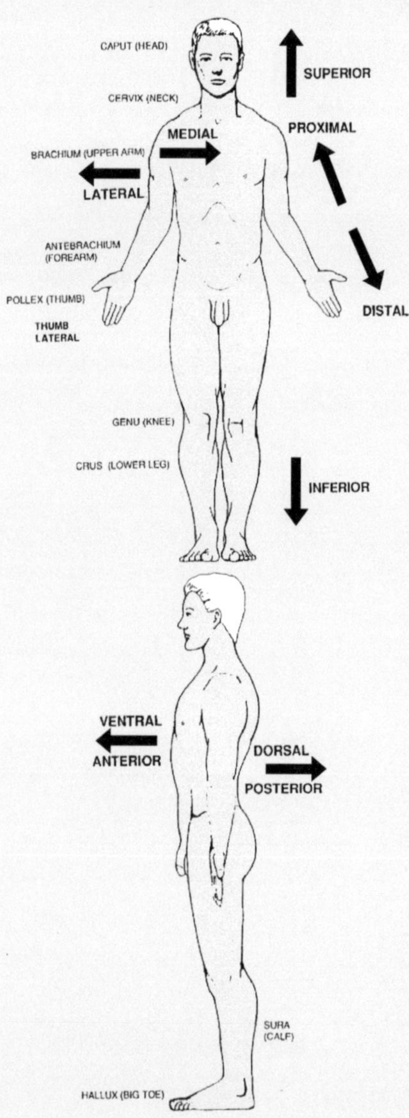
CAPUT (HEAD)
SUPERIOR
CERVIX (NECK)
MEDIAL
PROXIMAL
BRACHIUM (UPPER ARM)
LATERAL
ANTEBRACHIUM
(FOREARM)
POLLEX (THUMB)
THUMB
LATERAL
DISTAL
GENU (KNEE)
CRUS (LOWER LEG)
INFERIOR
VENTRAL
ANTERIOR
DORSAL
POSTERIOR
SURA
(CALF)
HALLUX (BIG TOE)

Anatomical Movements - Upper limb & shoulder

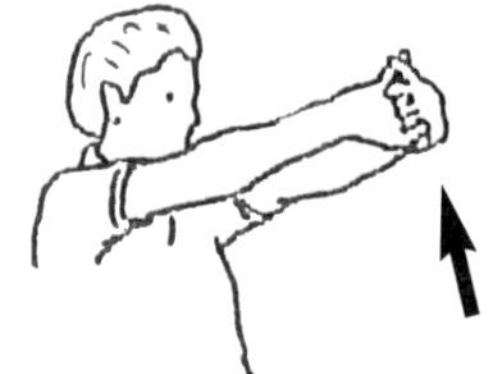

arm extension in sagittal plane / shoulder movement

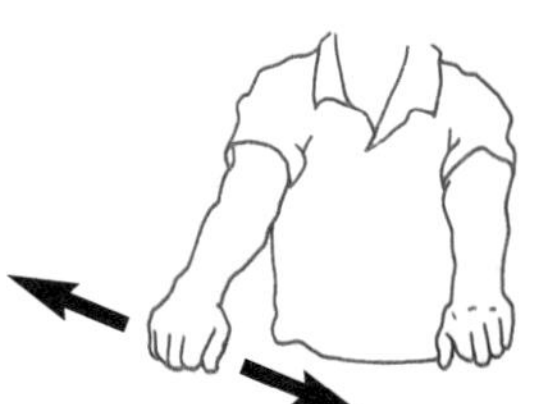

arm abduction -away from median plane / adduction-towards the median plane -shoulder movement

shoulder extension in the sagittal plane

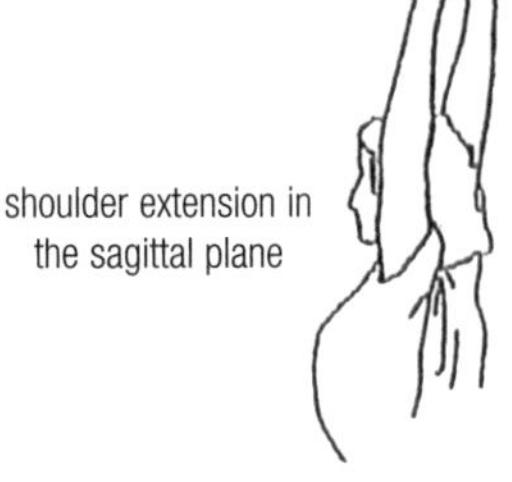

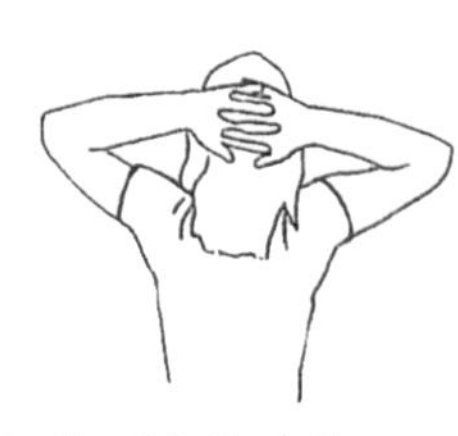

shoulder abduction in the coronal plane (with elbow flexion)

shoulder elevation
- reverse movement shoulder depression
shoulder movement

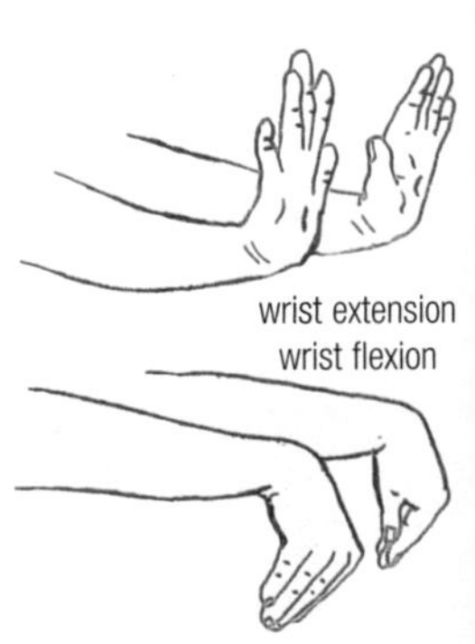

wrist extension
wrist flexion

arm/shoulder movements in the coronal plane commencing from adduction abduction to extension

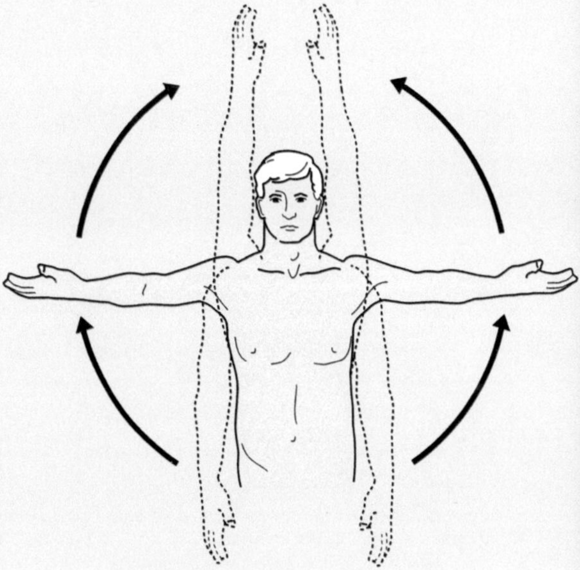

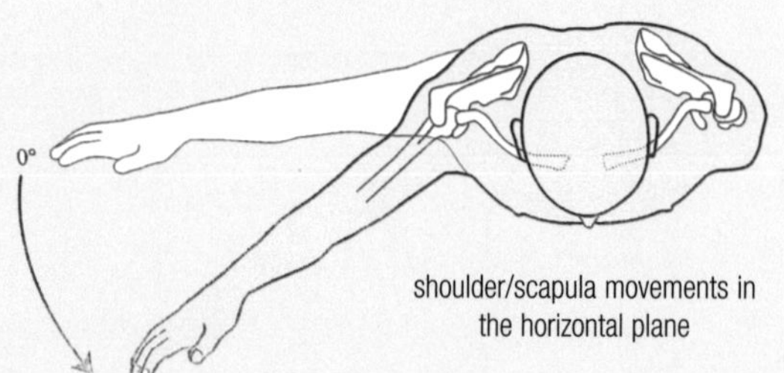

shoulder/scapula movements in the horizontal plane

Anatomical Movements - Head & Neck

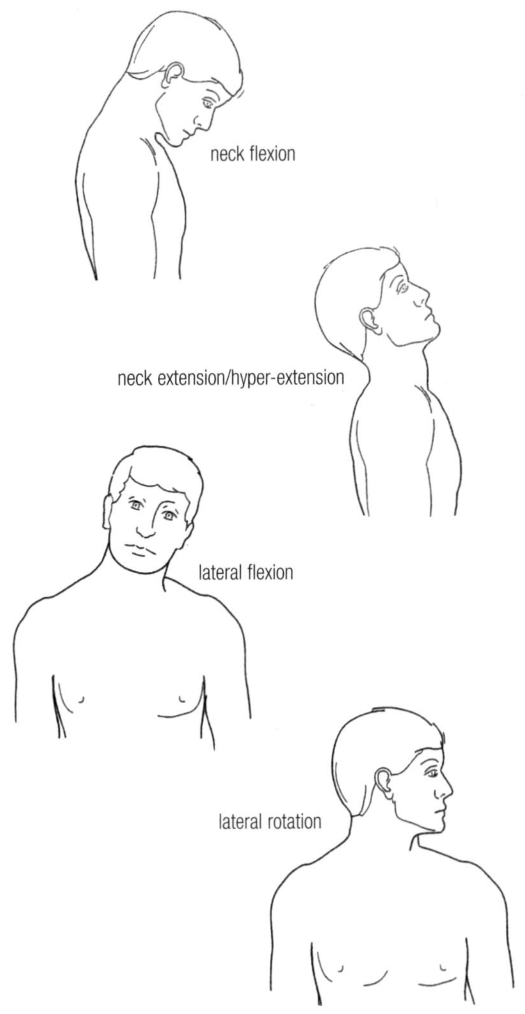

note: extension of the neck is in the normal anatomical position

Anatomical Movements - Back

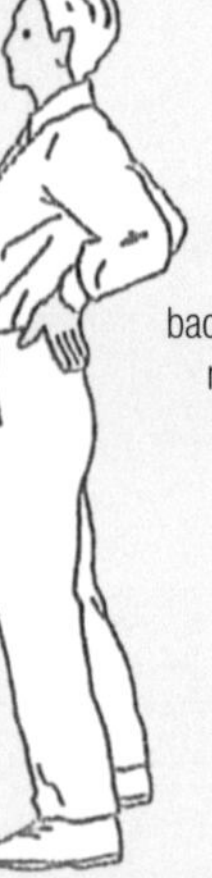

back extension / hyperextension
note the back muscles are
contracting

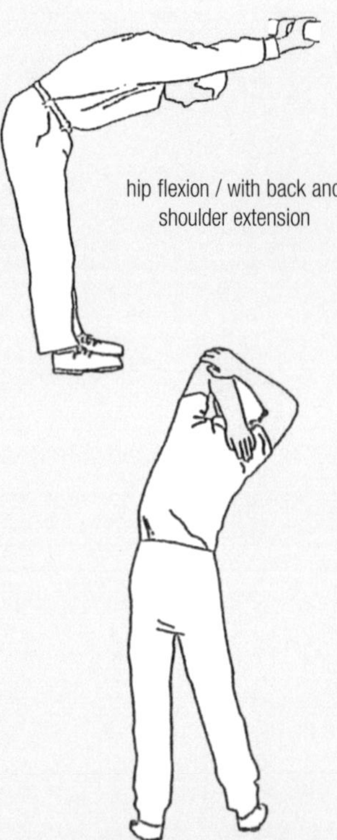

hip flexion / with back and
shoulder extension

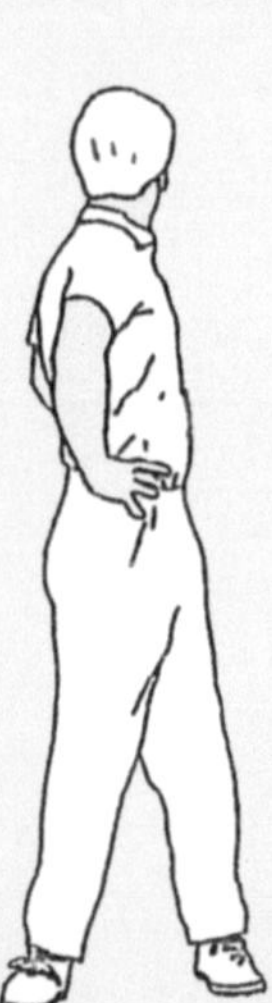

back rotation

back lateral flexion shoulder
extension and elbow flexion

Anatomical Movements - Lower limb & Hip

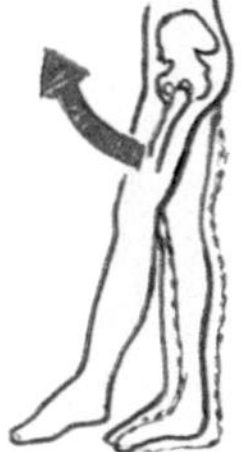

Hip flexion

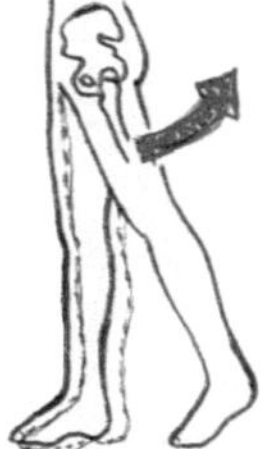

Hip extension

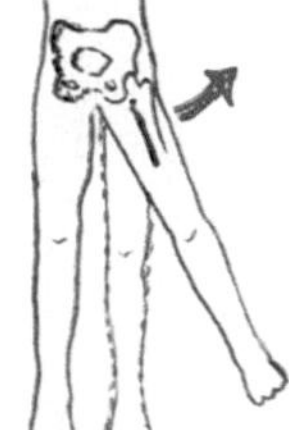

Hip abduction

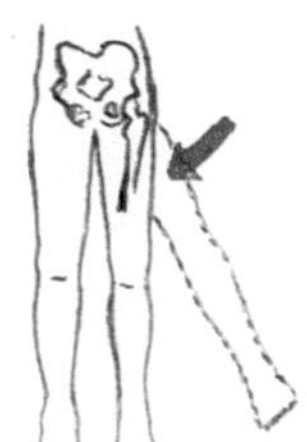

Hip adduction

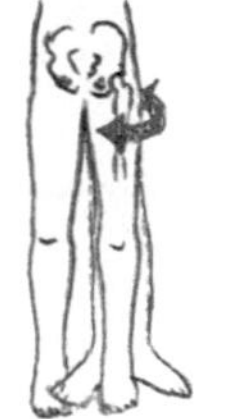

Hip lateral and medial rotation

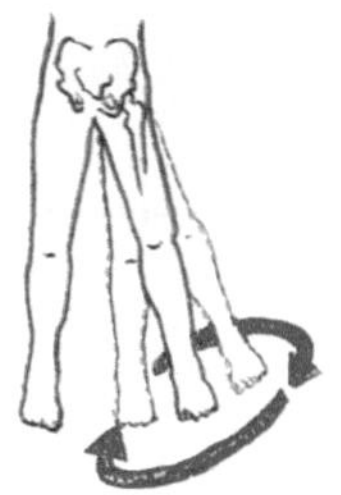

Hip circumduction

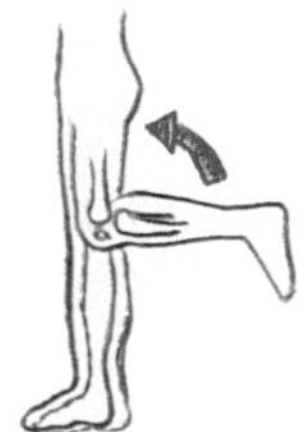

Knee flexion

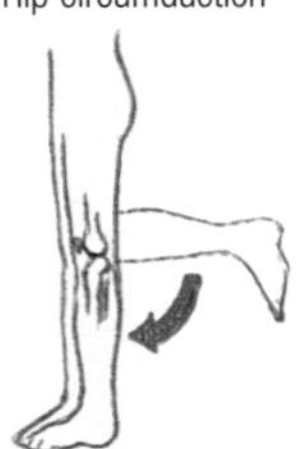

Knee extension

Anatomical Movements - Foot & hand

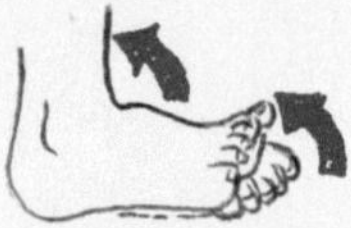

Foot dorsiflexion

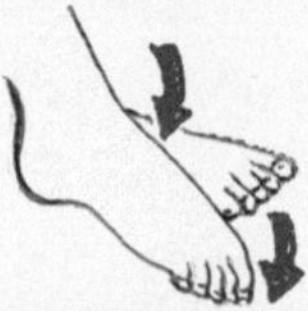

Foot plantar flexion

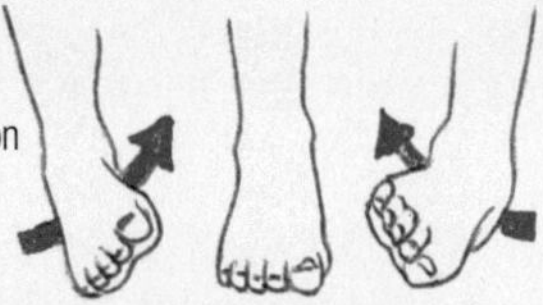

Foot inversion

Foot eversion

Foot normal position

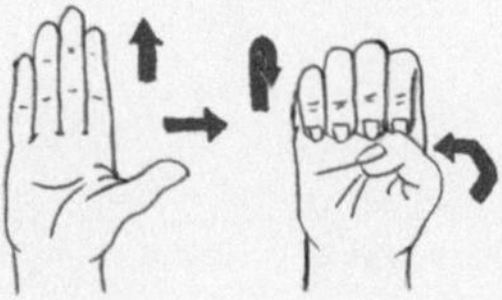

Fingers extension

Fingers flexion

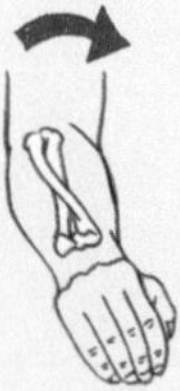

Forearm pronation

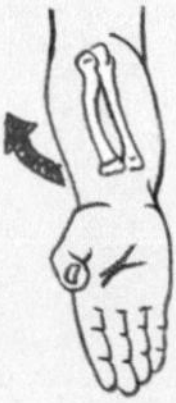

Forearm supination

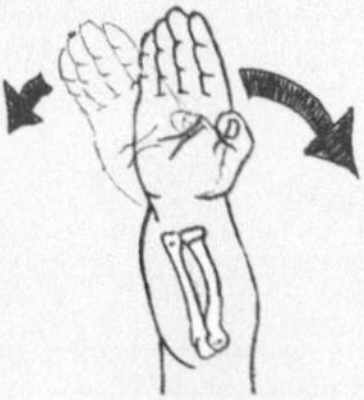

Hand deviation
radial/laterally
ulna/medially

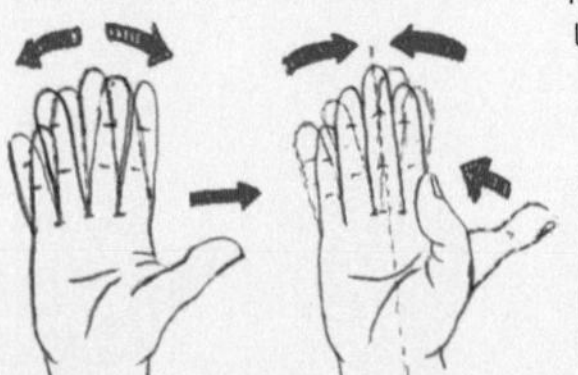

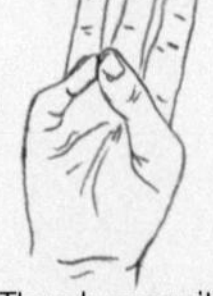

Fingers abduction

Fingers adduction

Thumb opposition

Foot Movements

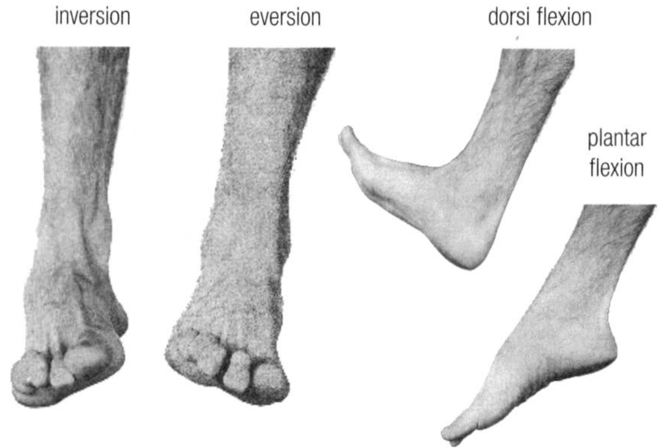

Hand Movements & Grips

The hand & wrist may be involved in a huge range of different grips & fine specialized movements calling upon a combination of muscles to allow for the precision of the actions.

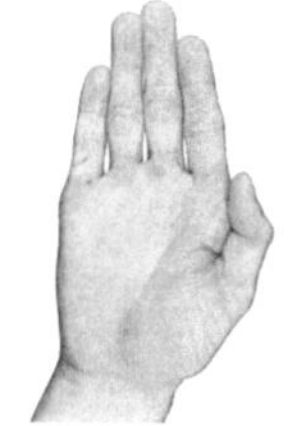

Finger thumb adduction
Dorsal Interossei

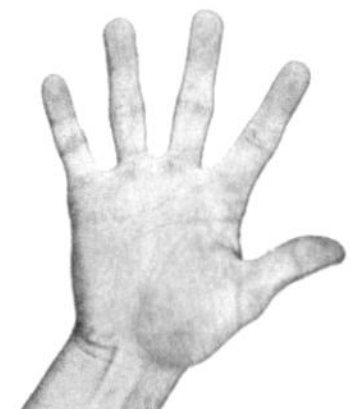

Finger thumb abduction
Palmar Interossei

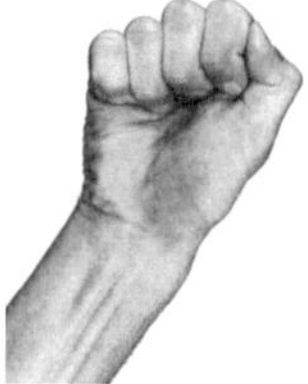

Finger thumb flexion
FDP, FPL

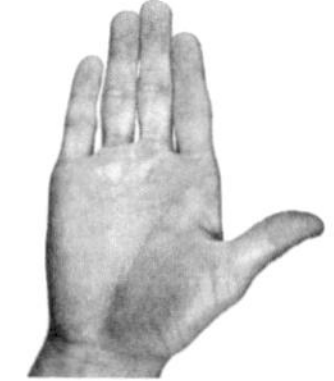

Finger thumb extension ant. dorso-lat *(anat snuff box) ED, EP*

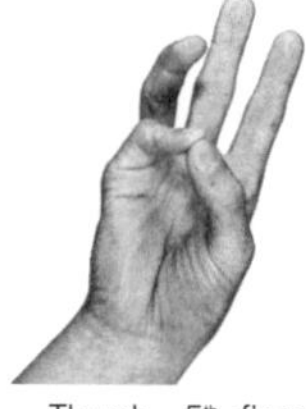

Thumb - 5th finger opposition *TE, HE, OP*

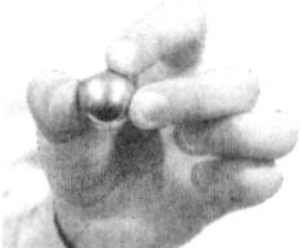

Opposition/flexion Carpal curve for precision grip

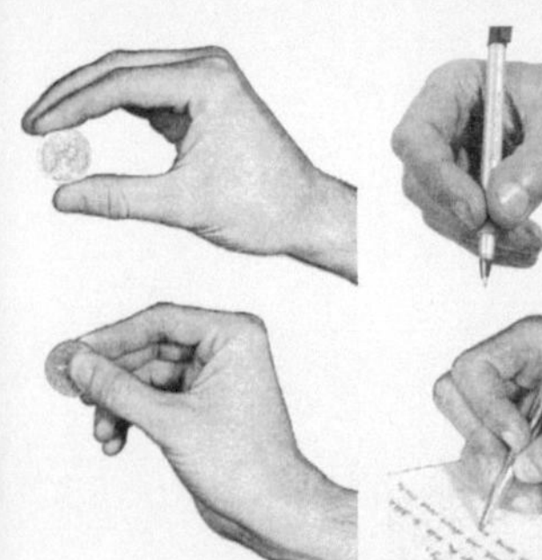

Thumb index – precision grip *TE, HE, OP*

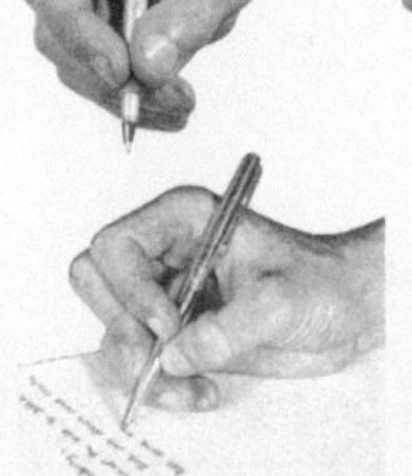

Thumb fingers - ± intrinsic hand muscles writing grip - precision *interossei*

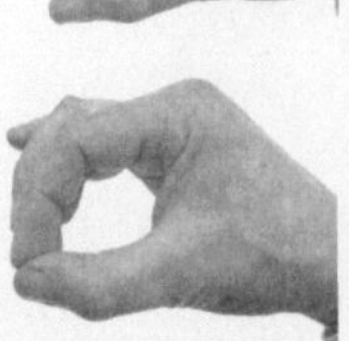

Open grip, Pinch lat.

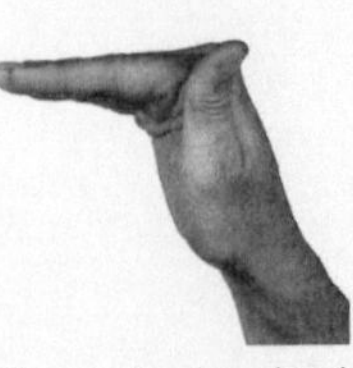

Finger extension - hand flexion *Lumbricles*

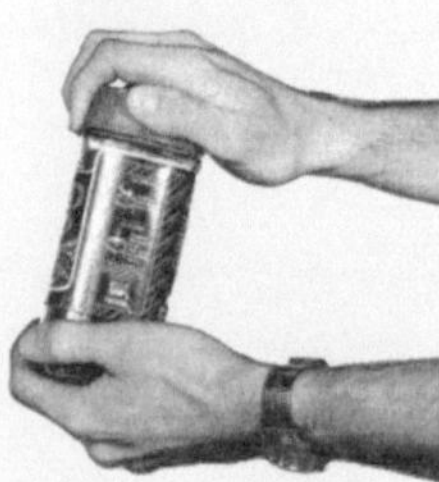

Hands coordinate in 2 handed procedures – unscrewing

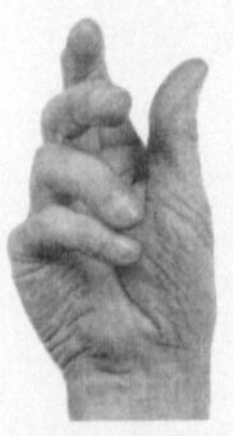

Power grips making use of friction - finger tips, PB HE+ TE for additional grip also boney curves - carpal curve shape of the phalanges

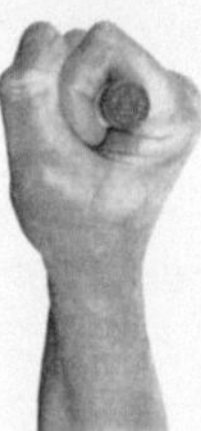

Practical holds demonstrating power grip variations

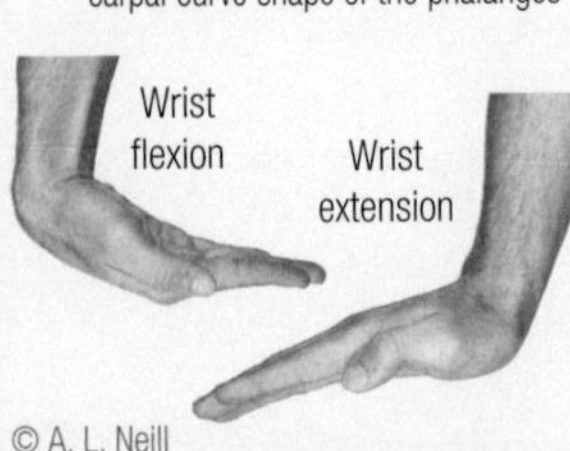

Wrist flexion

Wrist extension

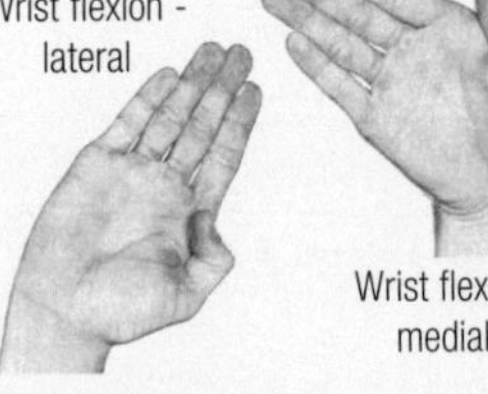

Wrist flexion - lateral

Wrist flexion medial

Hand Measurements

Measurements derived from the hand are part of the anthropomorphic measurements (measurements based upon human anatomy). They are helpful to the anatomist as they allow for rough clinical evaluations of surface anatomy w/o having to resort to more complex instruments –

Some other useful measurements have also been included.

9 of these measurements are included in the Vitruvian man.

cubit = 18 ins = 6 palms = elbow to fingertips = forearm + hand

digit < finger = fingertip (1)

ell = 45 ins = 15 palms = arm + body to shoulder

fathom = 72 ins = height

finger = width of finger (2)

foot = length of the shod foot, (longer than the bare foot)

hand = 4 fingers knuckle to knuckle = 4 ins (3)

inch = 25.4 mm = 1/12 part of … a foot
= thumb (i.e. width of at the nail base)

palm = 4 digits =3 inches =7.63cm (4)

shaftment = 2 palms = fist + outstretched thumb (5)

span = 3 palms = ½ cubit = extended hand (6)

yard = 12 palms = 36ins = arm + half body width

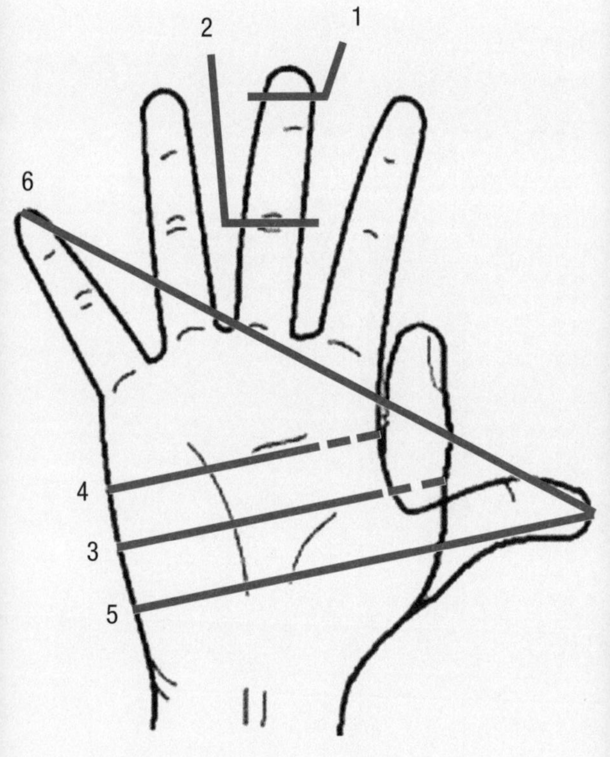
1
2
6
4
3
5

Proportions & forms of human measurement

Anthropic measurements = measurements based on human anatomy or behaviour
subset - Anthropomorphic measurements = measurements based upon human anatomy
measurements from the Vitruvian man include 9 basic anthropomorphic measurements included here are those based on height and arm span

Because of variation in heights and sizes these are hard to standardize but for the anatomist and clinician they provide a rough guide as to the normal proportions of the human body.

1/10 height	Face hairline - chin base	
1/8 height	elbow - axilla	arm
1/6 height	foot	neck - hairline
1/4 height	shoulder width	arm length
1/2 height	arm + half body	
height	arm span	4 cubits 1 pace
1/3 face	ear	hairline -eyebrows

1/10 height	Hand wrist –fingertip	
1/8 height		9 ins
1/6 height		1 ft
1/4 height		18 ins
1/2 height		3ft yard
height	24 palms 18 handbreadths	6ft fathom
1/3 face		

Human face proportions

The face varies greatly from person to person and certain races have specific characteristics – however in most cases the proportions of the major features are similar so the following is a guide to the standard proportions, which remain constant with age.

A common rule is that many of the features can be described in thumb lengths (T).

T = the length of the thumb from the tip to the MCP jt.

	Human face proportions
Chin	Chin to the root of the nose = **T**
Ear	Tip at the level of the Glabella = eyebrows Lobe at the level of the root of the nose = nasion. Length of ear = **T** Distance from the lobe to the angle of the jaw = ½ **T**
Eye	Distance b/n the eyes = **E** width of each eye = length of dorsum of the nose = width of the base of the nose
Mouth	Width of the mouth = distance b/n the Irises of the eyes = **M**
Hairline	If not receding - Glabella (eyebrows) to the hairline = **T**
Head	Up to 12- 13% of the height
Jaw line / angle	Midway b/n the nasion and the chin
Nose	Nose to the Glabella = **T** Width of the nose = distance b/n the eyes = the width of the eyes = **E**

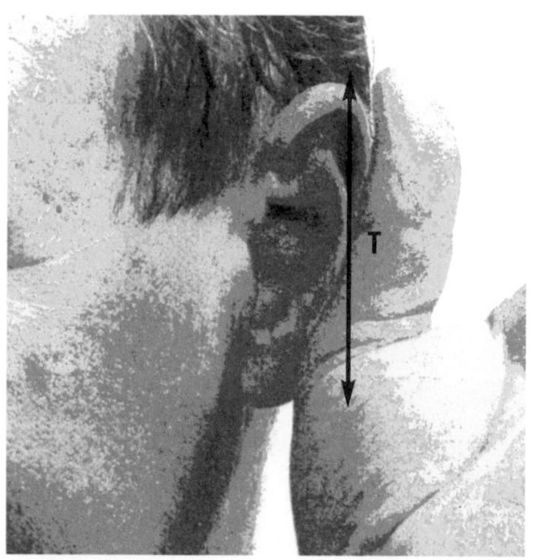
T

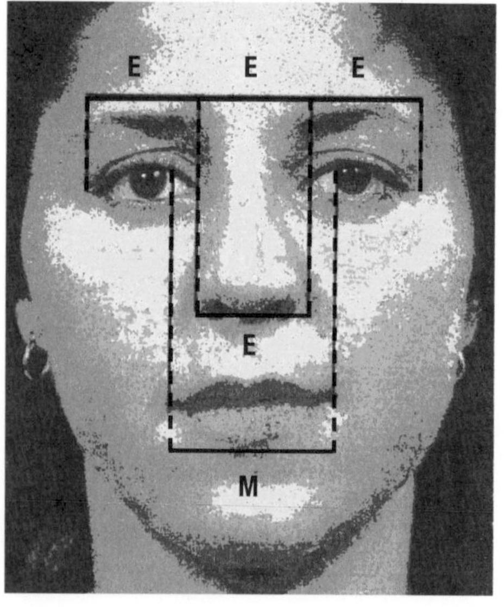
E
E
E
E
M

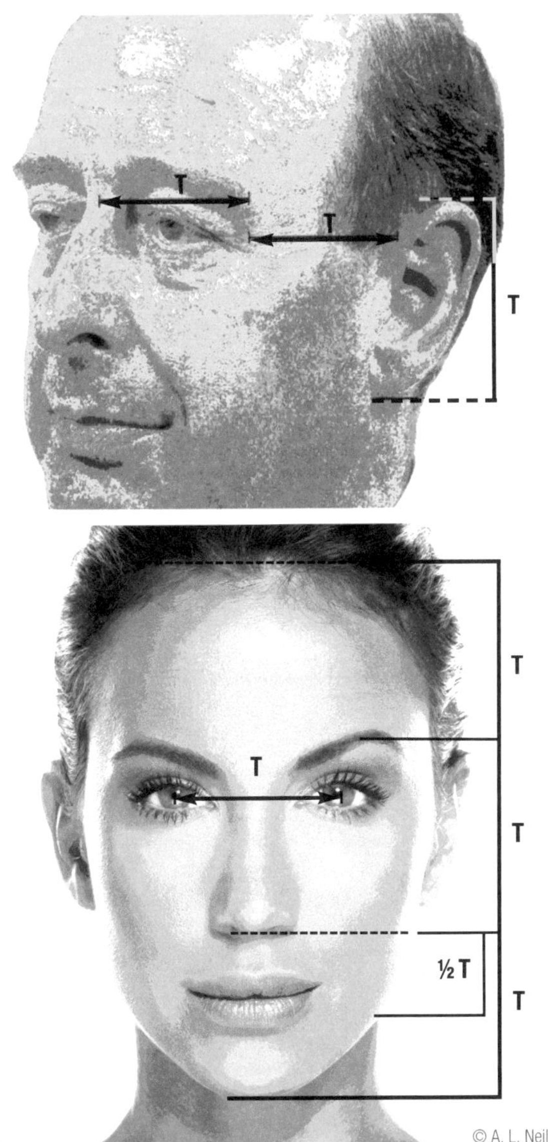
T
T
T
T
T
T
½ T
T

Proportions in the human body – b/n baby & adult

As the baby must be born with a view to increasing in size including: weight, length & breadth – and to changing functions including: maturity, mobility & independence certain features must be more advanced at birth than others, leading to changes in the proportions of those parts. For example the NS is almost completely developed at birth, but the limbs are not.

	Baby	Adult
Eye level	60% length of the face	50% face
Splanchocranium (facial skeleton)	50% face	68% face
Head	25% of height	13% of height
Midpoint of height / centre of gravity	Umbilicus	Pubis
Legs	33% height	50% height
Arms (fingertip to shoulder)	40% height	40% height

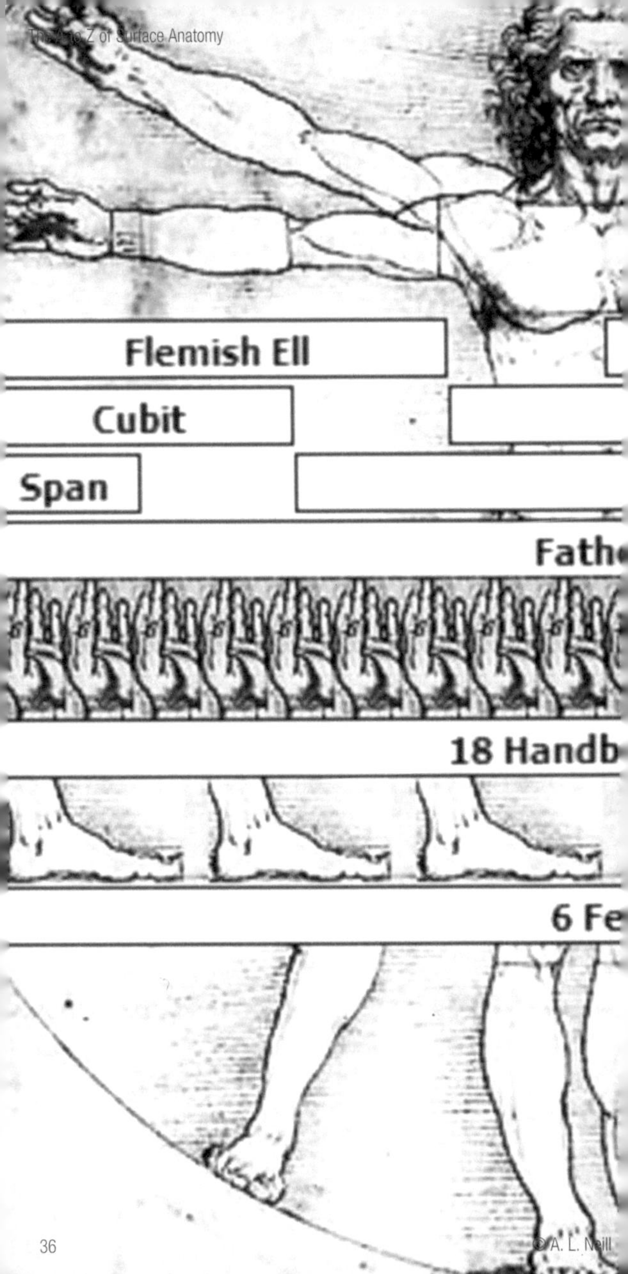
Flemish Ell
Cubit
Span
Fath
18 Handb
6 Fe

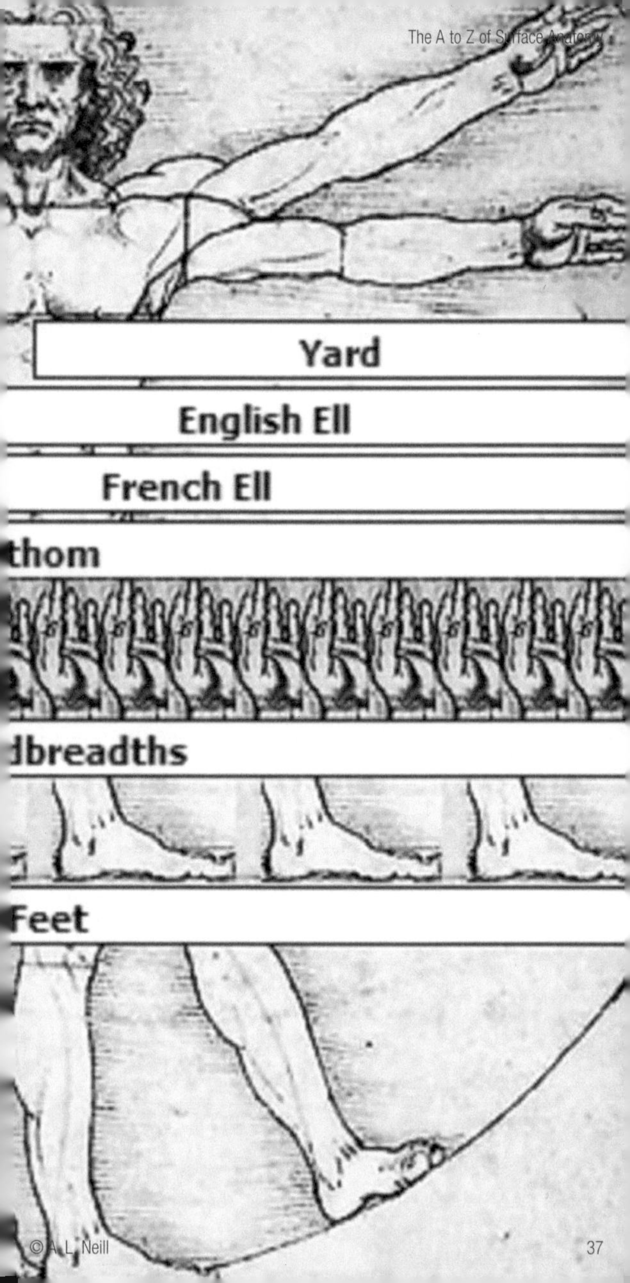
Yard
English Ell
French Ell
thom
dbreadths
Feet

Abdomen ant dermatomes

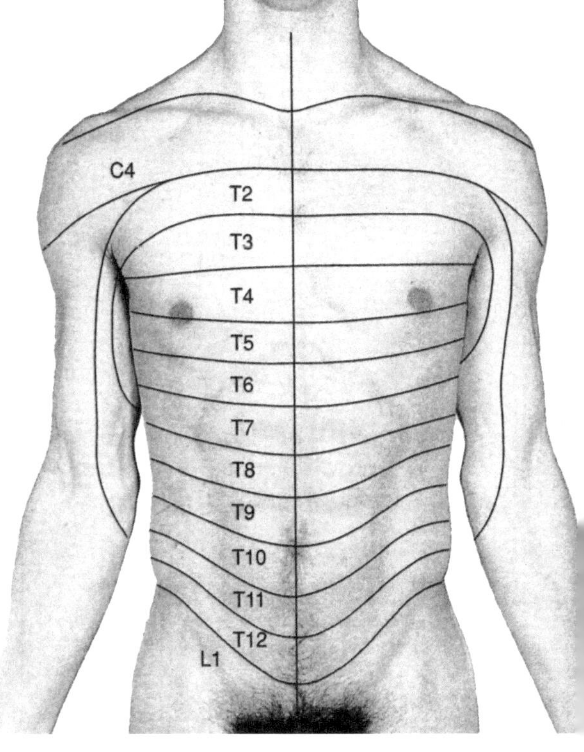

Abdomen post dermatomes

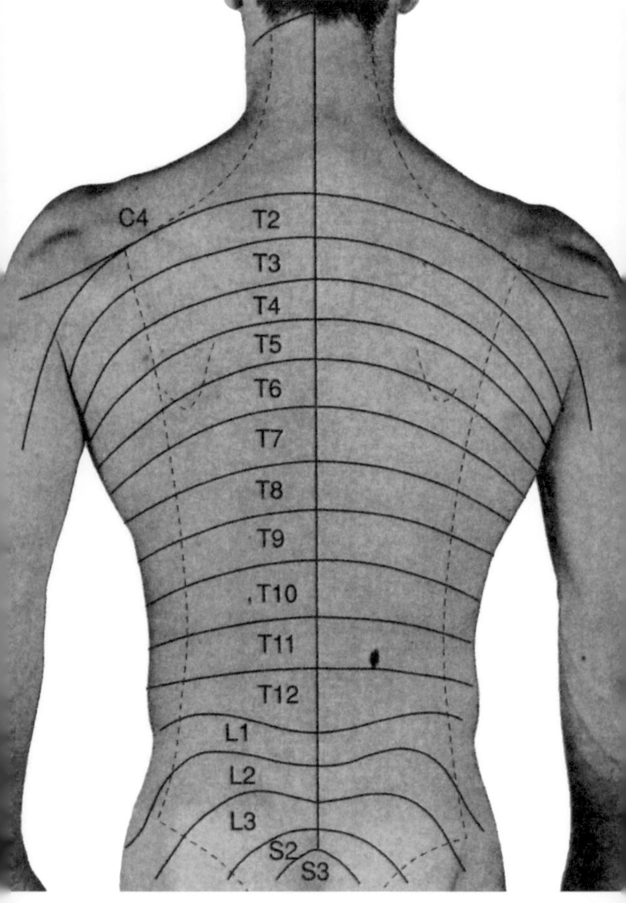

A B C D E F G H I J K L M N O P Q R S T U V W X Y Z

Anterior Abdominal Wall Muscles and Bones

Anterior view of the abdomen showing bones and muscles.

1 Sternum

2 Xiphoid process

3 3rd ICS

4-9 4th - 9th ribs

10 costal margin

11 1st intertendinous insertion (17)

12 2nd intertendinous segment – there are b/n 3-4 on each side (17)

13 linea alba

14 linea semilunaris L = left R = right

15 Quadratus Lumborum

16 inguinal ligament

17 Rectus Abdominus

18 iliac tubercle

19 iliac crest

20 ASIS

21 Pubic Symphysis

22 pubic tubercle

23 body of Pubis

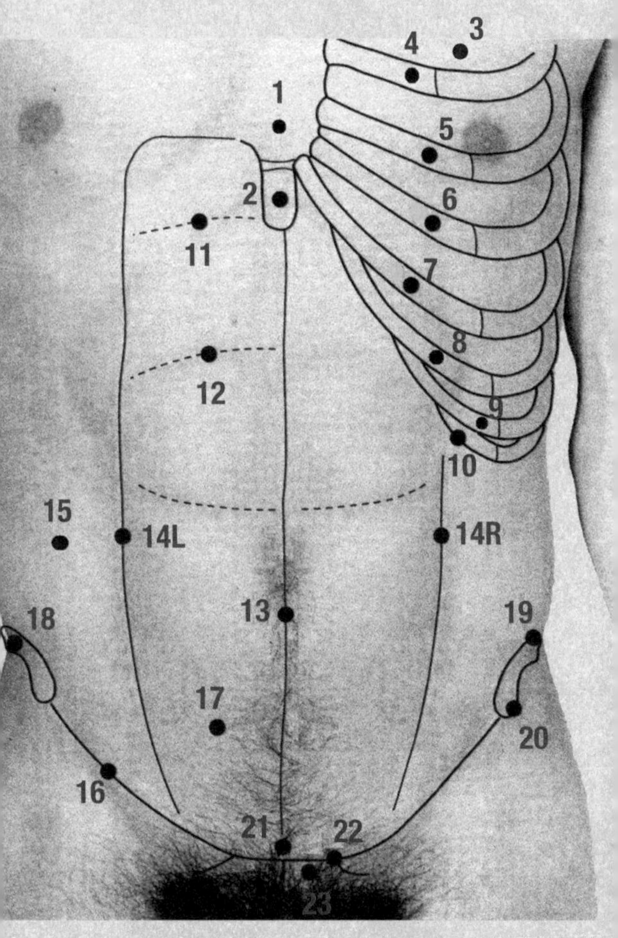
1
2
3
4
5
6
7
8
9
10
11
12
13
14L
14R
15
16
17
18
19
20
21
22
23

A

Abdominal Wall

GIT projection

B C D E F G H I J K L M N O P Q R S T U V W X Y Z

Anterior view of the abdomen showing the GIT projected.

1 Xiphisternum
2 oesophagus - *enters the abdomen at T10, L of the midline*
3 spleen
4 fundus of the stomach – *stomach fills the epigastric region, varies in size partially covered by the ribcage*
5 costochondral border
6 pyloris antrum ⇨ to pyloric sphincter
7 duodenum - first part - *begins R of midline below transpyloric plane near hepatic flexure of LI*
8 descending duodenum - second part
9 horizontal duodenum - third part
10 duodenojejenal flexure - *midline T12 subcostal plane*
11 terminal ileum - *in RIF*
12 appendix - *2/3 of line from ASIS to umbilicus*
13 caecum - *RIF closely assoc with appendix*
14 ascending colon - *retroperitoneal structure*
15 transverse colon - *attached to mesentery*
16 splenic flexure
17 descending colon - *retroperitoneal structure*
18 sigmoid colon - *attached to mesentery*
19 iliac tubercle
20 ASIS

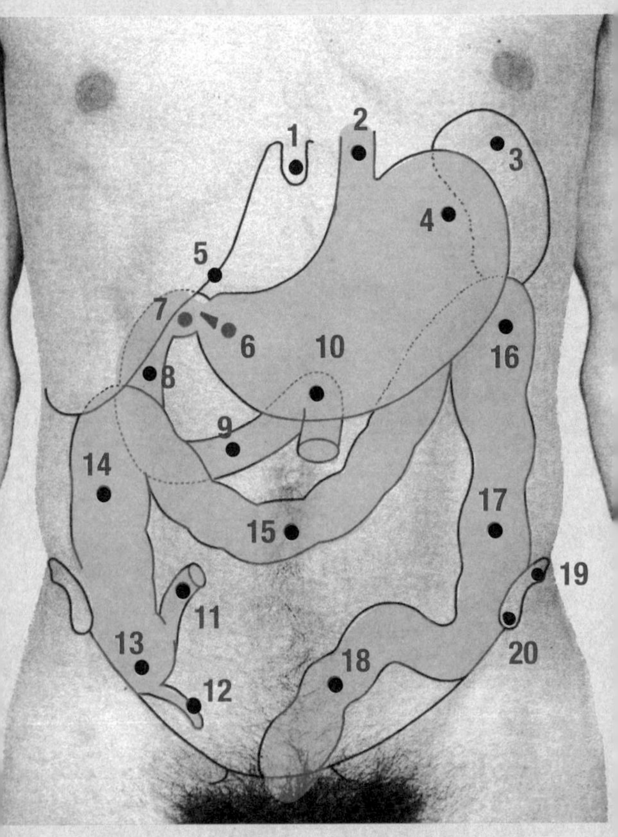

1
2
3
4
5
6
7
8
9
10
11
12
13
14
15
16
17
18
19
20

Abdominal Wall
non Alimentary structures projection

Anterior view of the abdomen showing the liver, pancreas & spleen.

1 liver - *fills the RH across to the epigastrium & above the CC to 4th ICS*

2 gall bladder - *MCL* ∩ *with the CC*

3 spleen - *post wall ribs 9-11*

4 pancreas - body - *stomach fills the epigastric region, varies in size partially covered by the ribcage*

5 pancreas - tail - *lodges in the hilum of the spleen*

6 pancreas - head - *lodges in the "C" of the duodenum*

7 duodenum -

8 aortic bifurcation - *ant. at the umbilicus - post. L4*

9 IVC - *midline to the R of the aorta - L5*

10 external iliac artery - *superior to inguinal lig at the MIP*

11 femoral artery - *inf to the inguinal lig*

12 inguinal ligament

13 ASIS

14 iliac tubercle

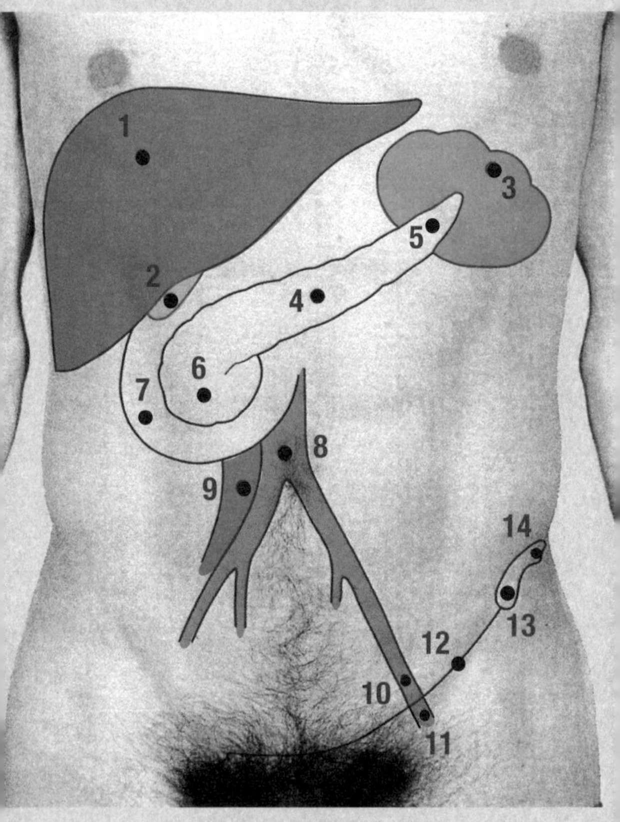
1
2
3
4
5
6
7
8
9
10
11
12
13
14

A B C D E F G H I J K L M N O P Q R S T U V W X Y Z

Abdominal Wall

Regions

Anterior view of the abdomen showing regions.

There are several ways to describe the regions of the Abdomen.

This commonly used schema divides the abdomen into 9 regions, based upon anatomical landmarks - numbered

Regions are coloured areas labelled with letters

1 Xiphisternum
2 midclavicular line (MCL) - *vertical line ½ way along the Clavicle*
3 transpyloric plane - *midway b/n Xiphisternum and umbilicus = L1 passes through pyloric sphincter and 1st part of the duodenum*
4 subcostal plane - *passes through L3*
5 transtubercular plane - *passes through L5*
6 Inguinal ligament
7 midinguinal point (MIP) - *intersection b/n MCL and inguinal lig*
8 anterior superior iliac spine = ASIS
9 iliac tubercle
10 7th rib - b= bone c = cartilage
11 MCL ∩ 9th rib
12 CC - *lower border of the ribs from the Xiphisternum around*
13 umbilicus - varies with age & weight approx. T10 dermatome

E = epigastrium - area b/n 3 & 12
H = hypochondrium - area b/n MCL 3 & 4 L = left & R = right
I = iliac region - area b/n MCL & 6 L= left & R = right
L = lumbar region - area b/n MCL & 4 & 5 L = left & R = right
P = pelvic area AKA suprapubic region - area below 5 above 6
U = umbilical region - area b/n MCLs 4 & 5

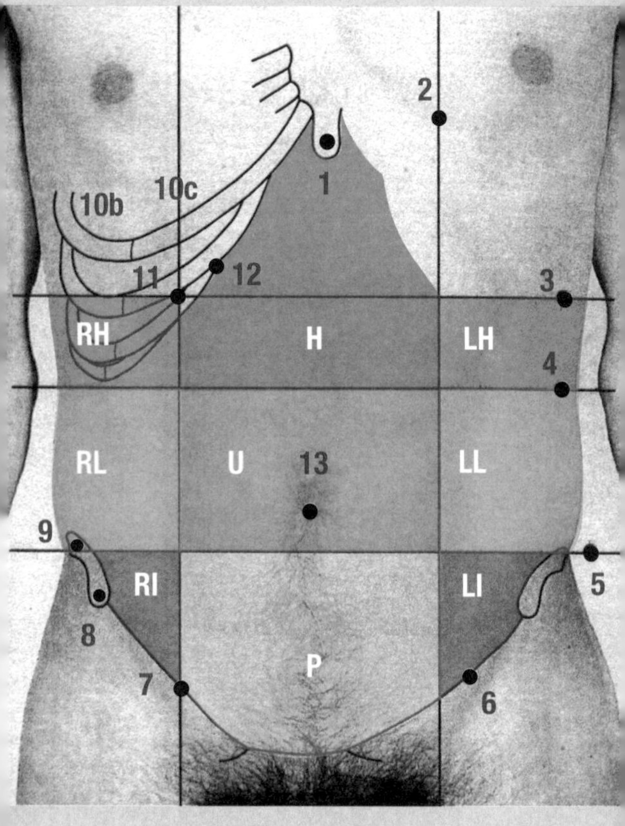

1
2
10c
10b
11
12
3
RH
H
LH
4
RL
U
13
LL
9
RI
LI
5
8
P
7
6

Abdominal Wall Incisions

Anterior view of the abdomen showing incision scars and their possible causes.

1 midline - *approach for upper GIT tract*

2 roof top - *approach for adrenals and kidneys*

3 renal - *may also be more posterior*

4 transverse - *to approach the pyloric sphincter / gastroduodenal junction, partic in infants*

5 laparoscopic point - *for access to the abdominal and pelvic organs*

6 peritoneal catheter insertion

7 suprapubic = *Pfannenstiel - approach for bladder uterus & adnexae Caesarean deliveries*

8 RIF - *approach for appendix*

9 subcostal - *approach for GB and liver*

10 paramedian - *superior to inguinal lig at the mid inguinal pt*

11 access pt for liver biopsy - *7th ICS axillary line*

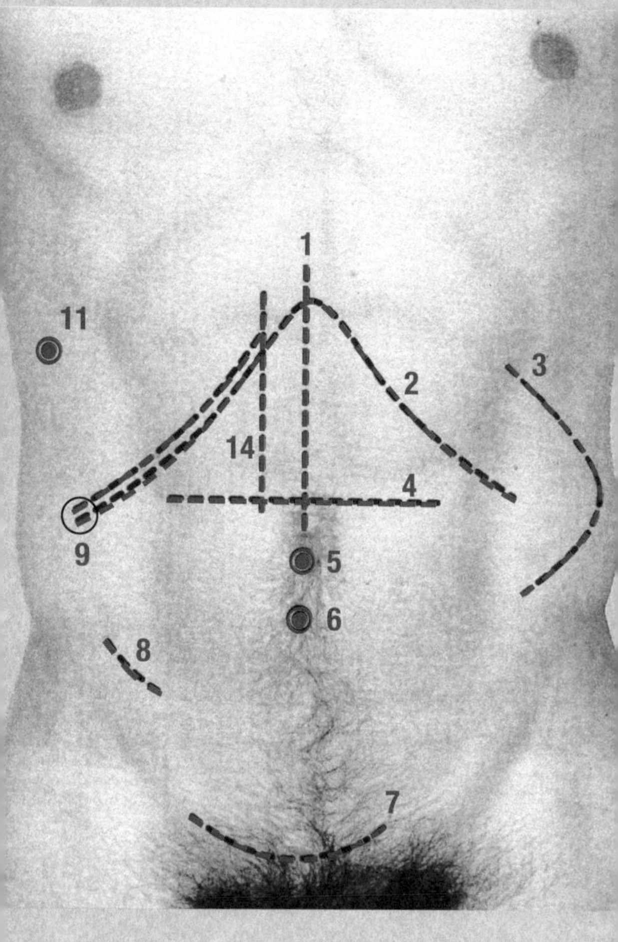
1
11
2
3
14
4
9
5
6
8
7

A B C D E F G H I J K L M N O P Q R S T U V W X Y Z

Ankle – tendons & retinacula

Lateral & medial views -

showing the tendons of the foot.

As with the hand & wrist, the muscles of the foot lie in the lower leg and tendons, encased in synovial sheaths, are restrained by a series of retinacula - strong fibrous bands

1 Ext. Hallicus longus
2a Tibialis ant.
2p Tibialis post.
3 Ext Digitorum longus
4b Peroneus brevis
4L Peroneus longus
4t Peroneus tertius
5 Flexor Hallicus longus
6 Flexor Digitorum longus
7 superior ext retinaculum
8 inferior ext. retinaculum l = lower / u = upper
9 flexor retinaculum l = lower / u = upper
10 superior retinaculum (lat)

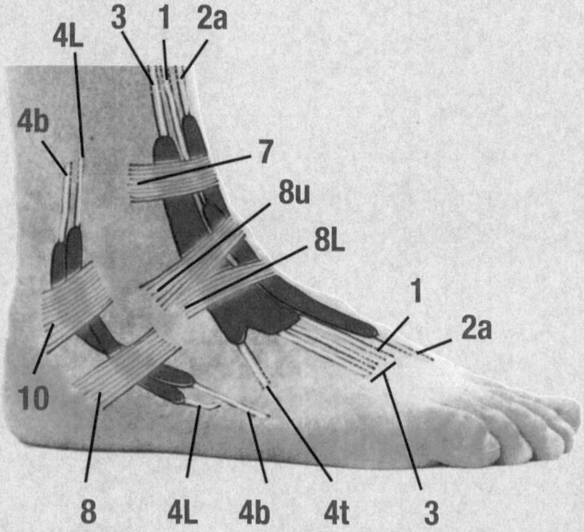

3
1
2a
4L
4b
7
8u
8L
1
2a
10
8
4L
4b
4t
3

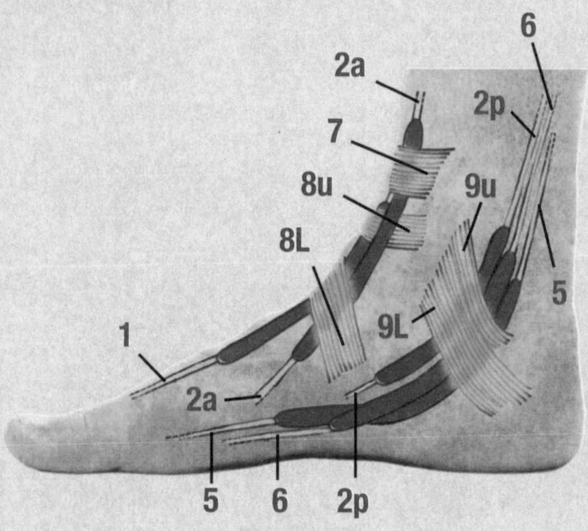
6
2a
2p
7
8u
9u
8L
5
9L
1
2a
5
6
2p

A B C D E F G H I J K L M N O P Q R S T U V W X Y Z

Aorta – Abdominal

Anterior view of the abdomen with projections of Aorta & Vena cavae.

1 aortic arch

2 descending / thoracic aorta -
gives off the intercostal arteries

3 site of aorta leaving the thorax and forming the
coeliac trunk – T12
beginning of the abdominal aorta

4 renal arteries L = left , R = right (slightly lower)

I transpyloric plane – midway b/n Xiphisternum and
umbilicus = L1/2

5 superior mesenteric artery

6 gonadal L = left , R = right (slightly lower)

II subcostal plane - passes through L3

7 inferior mesenteric artery

III intercristal plane = L4 site of the aortic bifurcation &...

8 formation of the Iliac arteries

IV transtubercular plane/intertubercular plane =
L5 b/n AIIS
site of formation of the...

9 9e = external iliac artery 9i = internal iliac

10 length of the abdominal aorta approx 10cm

11 11i = inferior vena cava 11s = superior vena cava

12 RA = right atrial wall

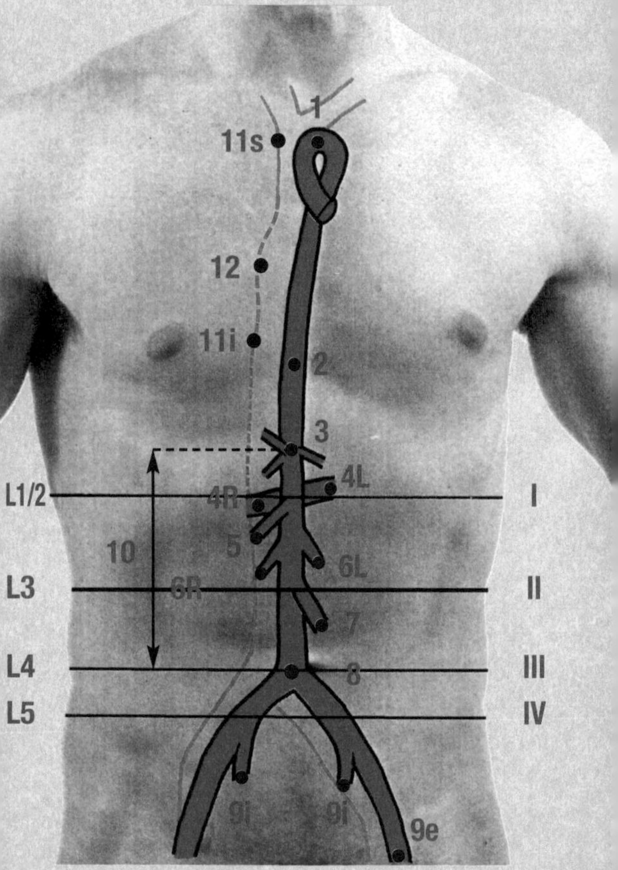

1
11s
12
11i
2
3
4L
L1/2
4R
I
10
5
6L
L3
6R
II
7
L4
8
III
L5
IV
9i
9i
9e

Arm

Muscles

Anterior view

abducted

medially rotated

flexed

1 FDS

2 Brachioradialis

3 Biceps

3L Biceps long head

3S Biceps short head + Coracobrachialis

4 Triceps

4L Triceps long head

4m triceps medial head

5 Brachialis

6 Deltoid

7 Latissumus dorsi

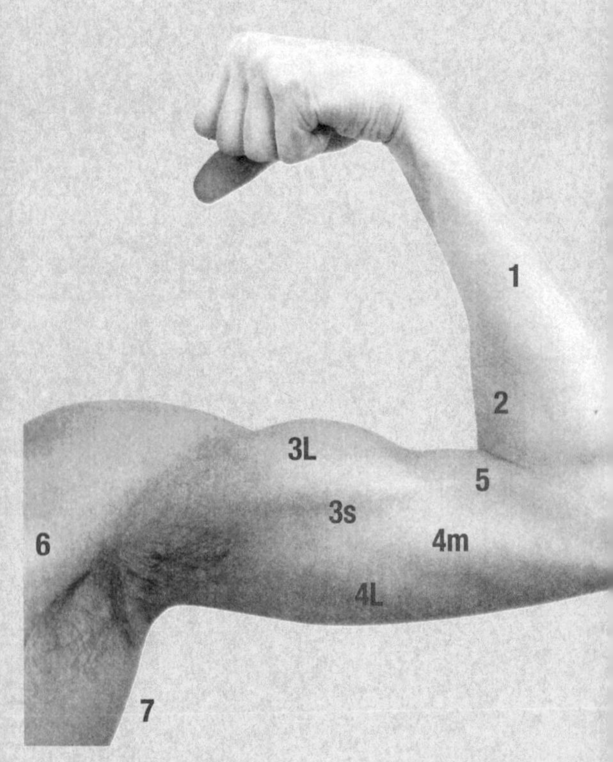
1
2
3L
5
3s
6
4m
4L
7

Axilla – Upper arm
Walls, Bones & Muscles

Lateral view extended abducted

Important site for the drainage of lymphatics of the upper limb and the breast

palpate here to determine swollen (cancerous) LNs from breast, chest and other thoracic structures

1 Biceps short head + Coracobrachialis
2 Triceps
3 Teres major with tendon of Latissimus Dorsi
4 Posterior axillary fold = Latissimus Dorsi
5 floor axilla – deep to this BP and Brachial BVs
6 Anterior axillary fold = Pectoralis major
7 Clavicle
8 muscle septum dividing Biceps & Triceps
9 Humerus
10 Scapula
11 Serratus anterior deep to the floor of the axilla & BP

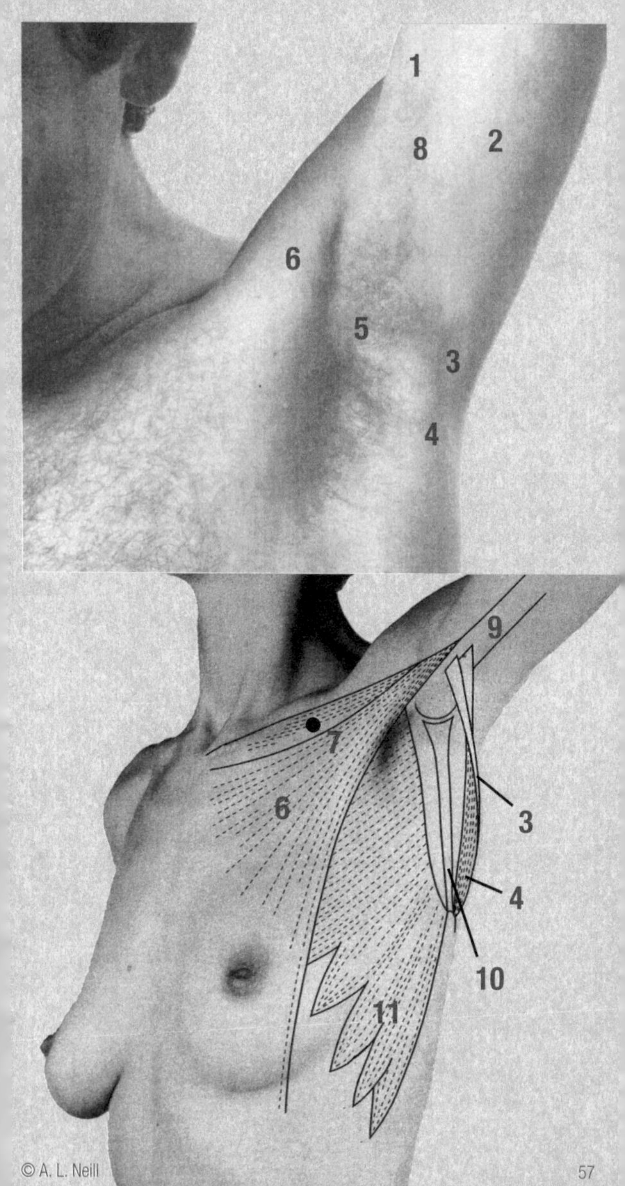
1
8
2
6
5
3
4
9
7
6
3
4
10
11

A B C D E F G H I J K L M N O P Q R S T U V W X Y Z

Axilla – Upper arm

Lymph nodes

Anterio-Lateral view –
extended –
abducted
laterally rotated

There are several different methods to name the LN groups. This naming is via location in the axilla. All groups are interconnected and palpated in breast examination. They drain the breast, UL and anterior chest wall - in particular the Virchow's group (6) may be the first sign of a silent cancer in the thorax.

1 Clavicle
2 Pectoralis Major m
3 Serratus Anterior m
4 Posterior axillary fold = tendon of Latissimus Dorsi m
5 Anterior axillary fold = Pectoralis Major m
6 Apical nodes – Virchow's Nodes – used as a sign of cancer
7 anterior nodes / pectoral nodes
8 medial nodes
9 posterior nodes
10 lateral nodes
10 +9+8+7 all drain to the highest apical nodes not shown here

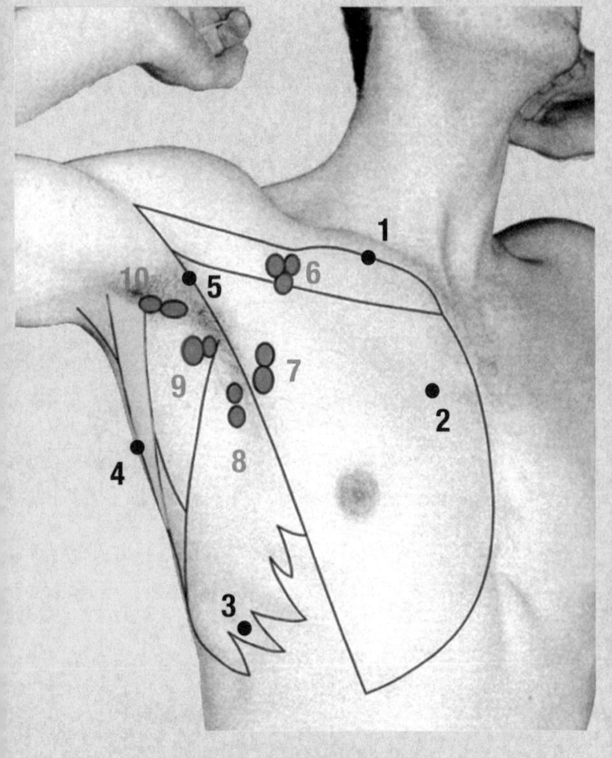
1
2
3
4
5
6
7
8
9
10

A B C D E F G H I J K L M N O P Q R S T U V W X Y Z

Back Lower = Trunk = posterior abdominal wall - kidneys, ribs, vertebral column

posterior view of the trunk = lower back

demonstrating access to retroperitoneal organs and VC -

1 limit of lung tissue

2 limit of pleura

3 10th rib (note moves down at least 2 vertebral segments)

4 intercristal plane – across the iliac crests and through the spine of L4 (sometimes b/n L3 & L4 site of lumbar puncture 11)

4s spine of L4

5 ureter 2cm lat of the VC

6 PIIS

7 Sacrum

8 iliac crest

9 incision site for .. L = lumbotomy (exposing kidney & adrenal)

n = nephrectomy (exposing kidney)

10 spleen

11 site of lumbar puncture b/n L2/3 or L3/4*

12 adrenal glands = suprarenal glands

**position for lumbar puncture is with a flexed spine in a non-erect patient (curled up and lying down)*

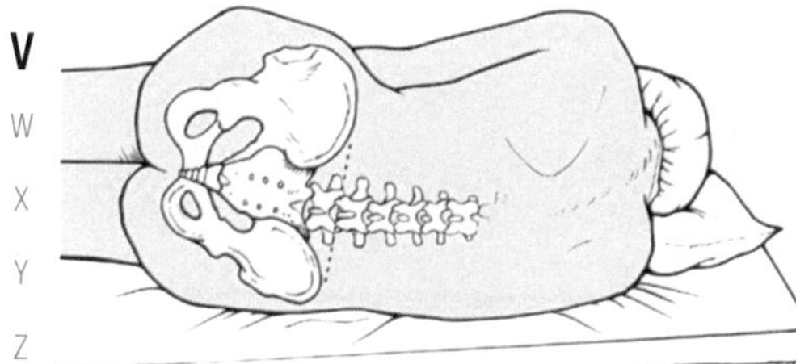

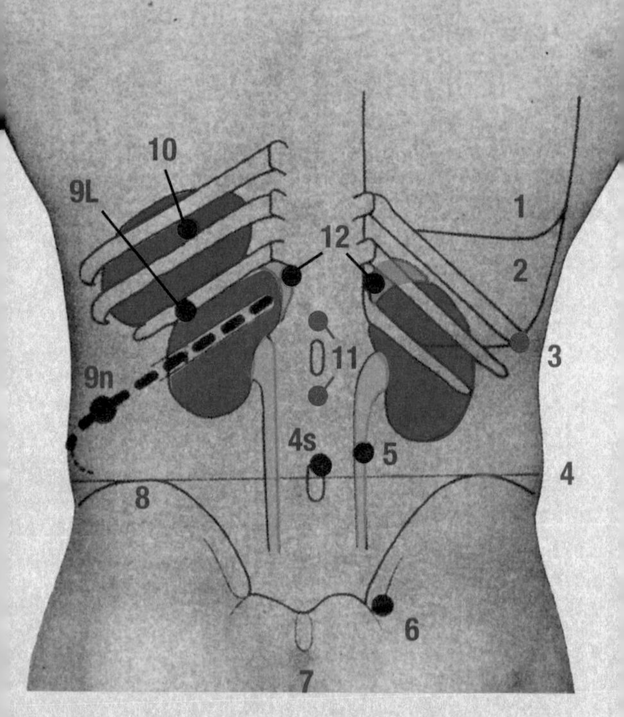
10
9L
1
12
2
11
3
9n
4s
5
4
8
6
7

Breast – female

Anterior view / extended / abducted

Arterial supply

The arterial BS of the Breast comes from 3 main sources which anastomose in the subareolar region or under the nipple and it is here that the venous drainage may be seen on the surface.

1. acromiothoracic artery
2. axillary artery – lateral thoracic branches
3. internal thoracic artery – anterior perforating branches

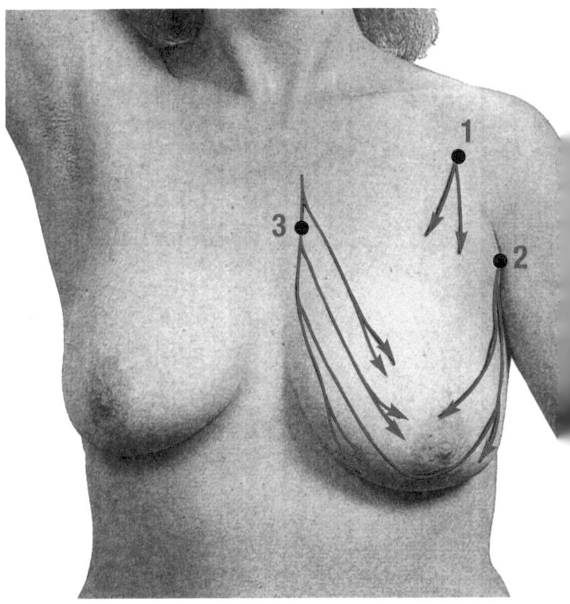

Lymphatic & venous drainage

The lymphatic drainage of the Breast goes mainly via the pectoral nodes (8) to the axilla along with the main venous drainage (9) but especially in the case of blockage to the main routes – lymphatic drainage may also go contralaterally (6) and even to the inguinal nodes (7).

4 supraclavicular nodes
5 nodes along the internal thoracic artery & vein
6 nodes along the contralateral internal thoracic vessels
7 lymphatics to abdomen & inguinal region
8 pectoral nodes
9 central / axillary and apical nodes

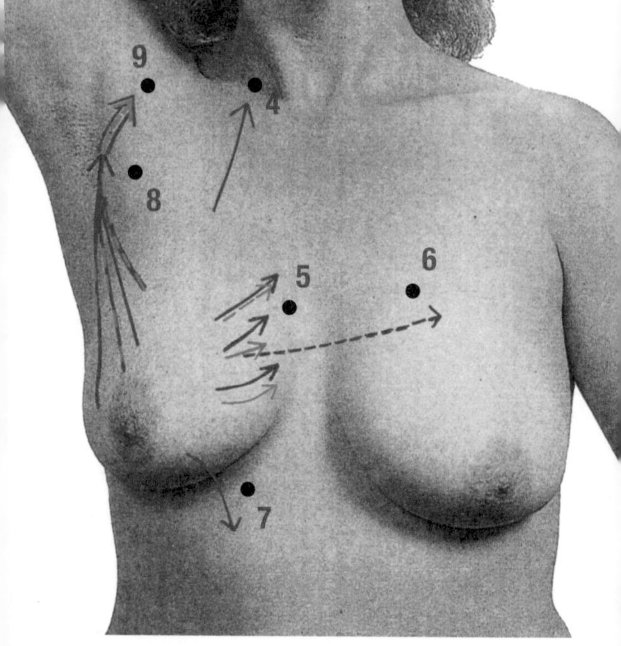

A B C D E F G H I J K L M N O P Q R S T U V W X Y Z

Chest Wall

Great Vessels

C *Anterior projection of the great vessels on the chest wall with rib cage.*

1-6 ribs
7 SVC
8 brachiocephalic venous trunks L & R
9 inominate artery = brachiocephalic
10 L common carotid
11 L subclavian artery
12 pulmonary trunk
13 ascending aorta and arch
14 IVC

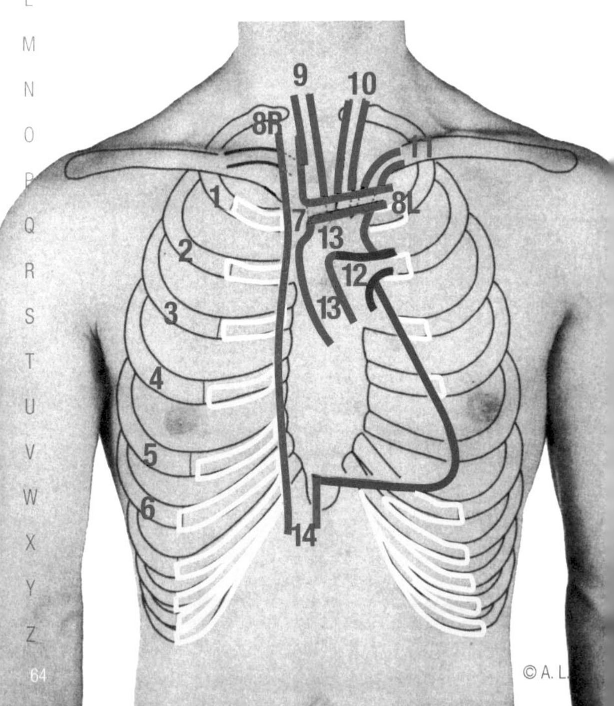

Chest Wall
Heart

Anterior projection of the heart and its chambers on the chest wall with rib cage.

1-6 ribs 1-6
7 aortic arch
8 auricle L & R
9 R atrium
10 coronary sulcus
11 ventricle L & R
12 AV sulcus anterior
13 apex

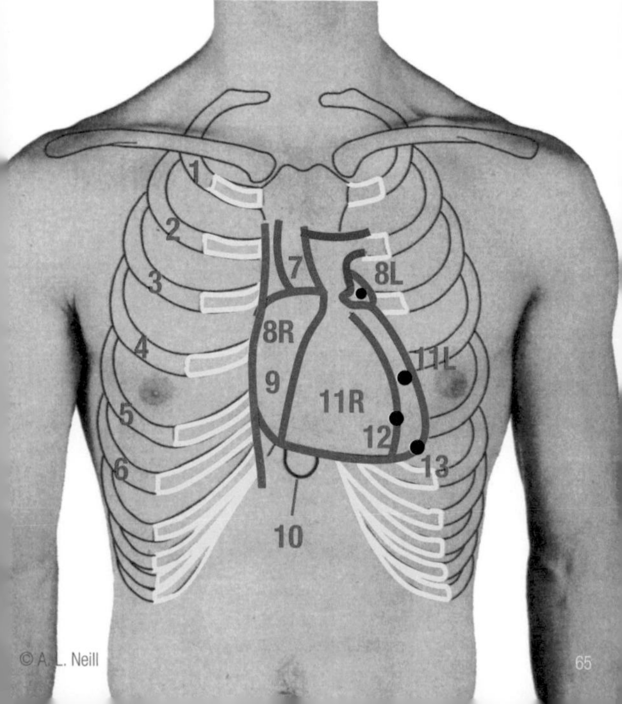

A B **C** D E F G H I J K L M N O P Q R S T U V W X Y Z

Chest Wall

Heart Valves & Heart Sounds

Anterior projection of the cardiac valves and the sites for auscultation great vessels on the chest wall with rib cage.

1-6 ribs

A site of auscultation

V site of valve

a = aortic valve

m = mitral valve

p = pulmonary valve

t = tricuspid valve

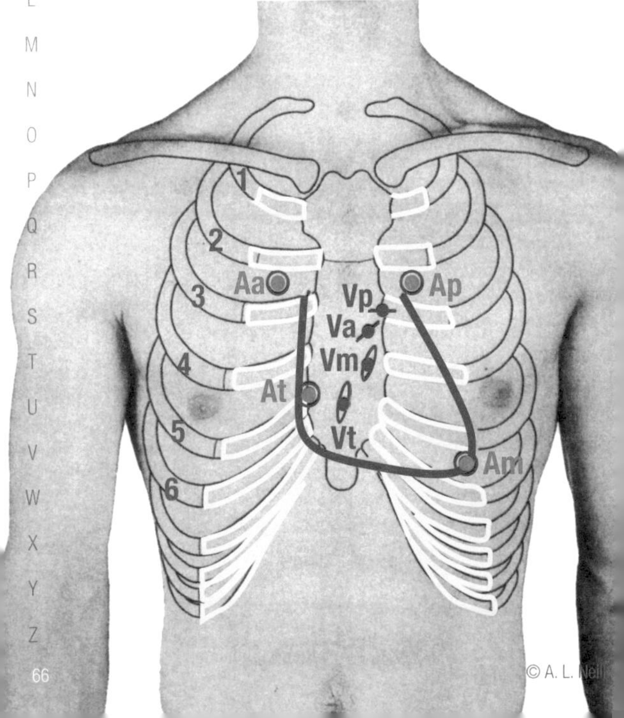

Chest Wall
Incisions

Anterior view of the chest showing incision scars & their possible causes.

1 midline - approach for Mediastinum
2 access point for ventricles - approach heart ventricles
3 access point for pericardial cavity - approach to drain pericardial sac
4 posterolateral thoracotomy - to approach via the bed of the 4th rib
5 posterolateral thoracotomy - to approach via the bed of the 5th rib
6 catheter insertion to the pleural sac - for drainage
7 thoracoabdominal incision

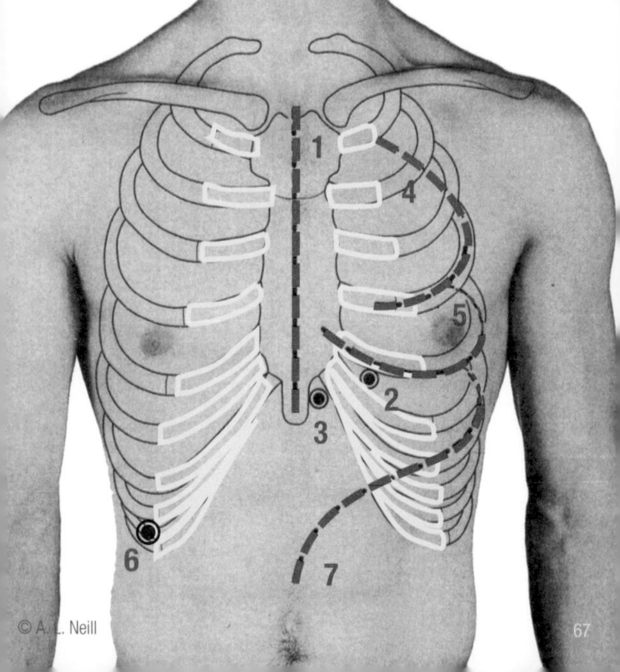

Chest Wall

Lungs & Pleura

Anterior view of the chest showing lung and pleural sac markings.

Note lungs come above the ribs anteriorly and there is a greater disparity b/n pleura and lungs in the ant. than post.

3 lobes on the R lung – additional fissure

2 lobes on the L lung – cardiac notch

1 Manubrium – has jts with rib 1 & Clavicle
2 outline of lungs
3 outline of parietal pleura
4 oblique fissure – lungs + visceral pleural makings
5 Sternum (1 + 5 = manubriosternum) anchors ribs 2-6 individually and the CC of ribs 7-10
6 6th rib
7 ribs 7-10 attached via CC to the Sternum
8 horizontal fissure – R side 4th ICS
9 cardiac notch – L side 4th ICS

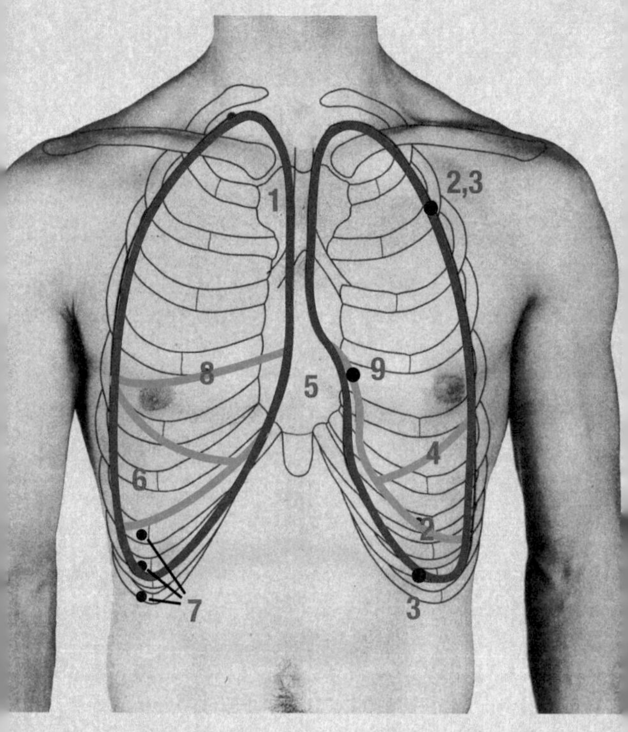
1
2,3
8
5
9
4
6
2
7
3

A B C D E F G H I J K L M N O P Q R S T U V W X Y Z

Chest Wall

Lungs & Pleura

Posterior view of the chest showing lung and pleural sac markings.

note lungs do not come above the ribs posteriorly

1 spinous process of T1 – attached to rib 1
2 outline of lungs
3 outline of parietal pleura
4 oblique fissure – lungs + visceral pleural makings
5 thoracoabdominal incision post.
6 6th rib
7 vertebra prominens – defn – most prominent spinous process (usually C7 rarely C6)
8 distance b/n spinous processes and lung pleural usually 2 fingers 2 ½ cm
9 floating ribs 11,12

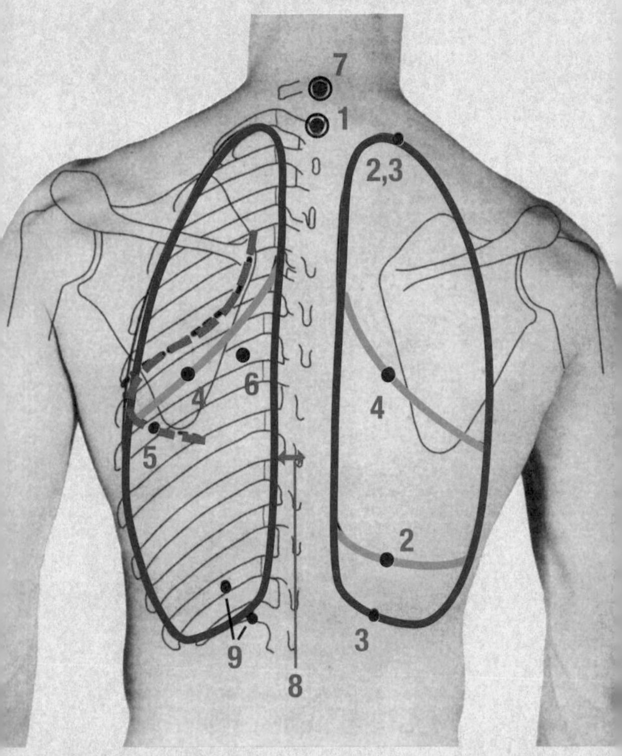
7
1
2,3
4
6
4
5
4
2
9
3
8

A B **C** D E F G H I J K L M N O P Q R S T U V W X Y Z

Cubital Fossa

Bones, Muscles and Vessels

Anterior views - deep to superficial

Clinically important area for accessing venous and arterial blood, testing reflexes and muscle strength in the upper limb - defn - the area b/n the Biceps & its aponeurosis & the muscles of the common flexor origin & Brachioradialis (anterior fossa of the ant of the elbow)

1 Humerus – anterior surface
2 epicondyles of Humerus l = lateral m = medial
3 Capitulum
4 head of Radius
5 bicipital tuberosity
6 coronoid process (of Ulna)
7 trochlea
8 interosseus membrane

9 Biceps a = aponeurosis
10 Brachioradialis
11 Flexor digitorum superficialis
12 common flexor origin
13 Pronator Teres
14 Brachialis

15 cephalic vein
16 median cubital vein
17 basilic vein
18 brachial artery
19 ulnar artery
20 radial artery

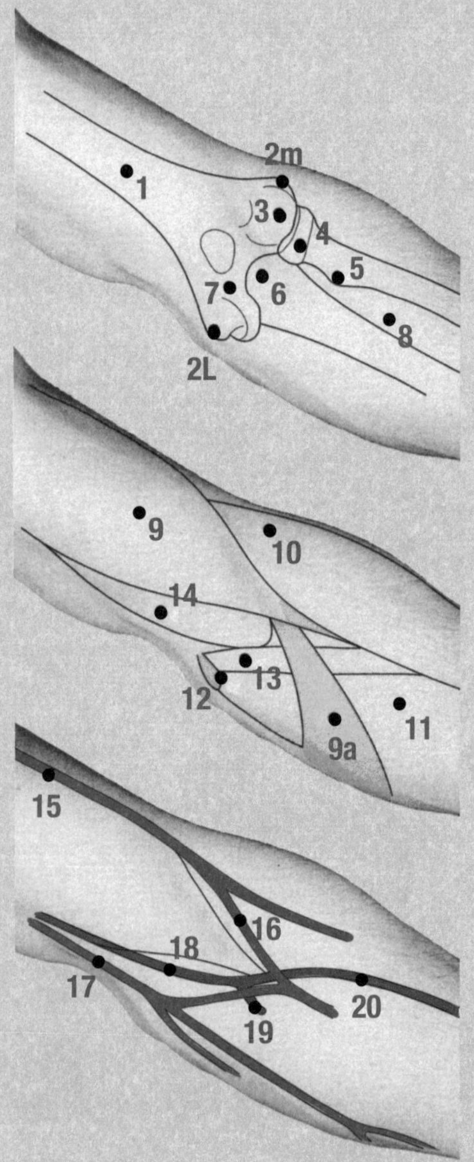
2m
1
3
4
5
7
6
2L
8
9
10
14
13
12
11
9a
15
16
18
17
20
19

Diaphragm + Gallbladder + Liver + Spleen

Anterior view

Expiration - Inspiration.

Diaphragm = a musculotendinous dome, dividing the thorax & abdomen, centrally flattened the L(4th ICS T10-11) > R (6th rib T12) – both in the MCL (through the nipple).

Up to 1 rib higher in the supine position and in the broad-chested.

Resting respiration - ± 1cm – but may vary up to 10cm.

Attached - ant. – to the Xiphisternum, costal margin
lat. - ribs 6-12
post. L1-3

contraction - flattens the dome shape –
pulls the IVC open
↑ abdominal P
↑ core strength
lowers & moves the Liver to the L
lowers & flattens the Spleen to the R

Both the Live r& Spleen are intimately related to the Diaphragm and the IVC and move as described.

1 Liver L = left R = right
p = ptosed (ie lowered in inspiration)
Liver edge palpable just below the CC on inspiration -

2 Gallbladder (9th CC) – divides the liver into the R & L functional ½

3 Spleen spans ribs 6-9 NAD – but in certain disease states partic parasitic infections - (malaria) may fill down to the LIF
p = ptosed (ie lowered in inspiration)

4 Diaphragm e =expiration position
i = inspiration position
n = neutral position

A B C D E F G H I J K L M N O P Q R S T U V W X Y Z

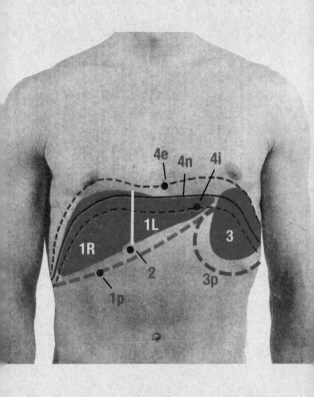

4e
4n
4i
1L
1R
3
2
1p
3p

Ear

External view of the ear and its components.

1 triangular fossa
2 helix
3 antihelix
4 tragus
5 EAM = external auditory meatus
6 antitragus
7 lobe
8 scapha
9 concha

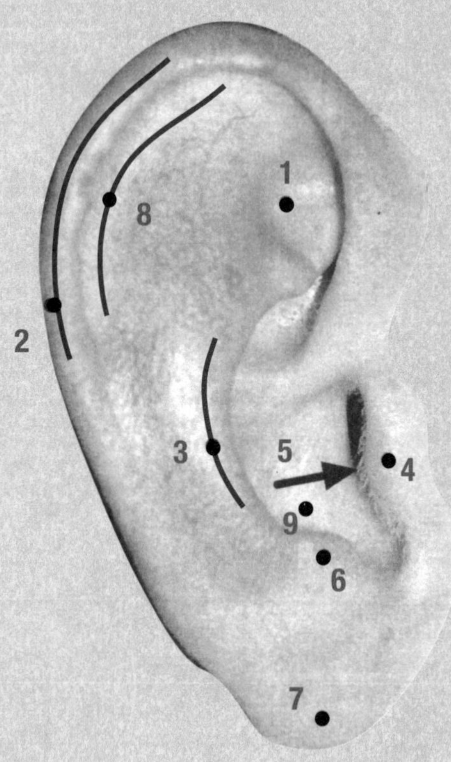
1
8
2
3
5
4
9
6
7

A B C D **E** F G H I J K L M N O P Q R S T U V W X Y Z

Eye

External view of the eye and its components

Anterior View - sulci increase with age

Eversion of the Lower Lid - can examine the conjunctiva & assess anaemia

Eversion of the Upper Lid - exposures the upper tarsal plate - cartilaginous support for the lid - & tarsal glands in allergies, & foreign bodies.

1 eyebrow
2 upper eyelid orbital part
3 palpebral sulcus i = inferior, s = superior
4 upper eyelid tarsal part
5 angle of the eye L = lateral m = medial in b/n the palpebral fissure 5f (where the upper & lower lids meet)
6 nasal jugal sulcus
7 eyelashes
8 malar sulcus = lateral sulcus
9 iris
10 pupil

11 sclera = bulbar conjunctiva
12 papilla lacrimalis (raised surface)
13 punctum lacrimale (opening for tear duct)
14c caruncula lacrimalis = lacrimal caruncle - (tear duct)
14s sac for lacrimal gland
15 lacus lacrimalis
16 plica semilunaris
17 palpebral conjunctiva
18 lower lid margins (ant & post)
19 tarsal glands and openings
20 inf fornix of the conjunctiva

21 branches of posterior conjunctival arteries
22 tarsal plate (lower is much thinner 22L)
23 upper lid margins (ant & post)

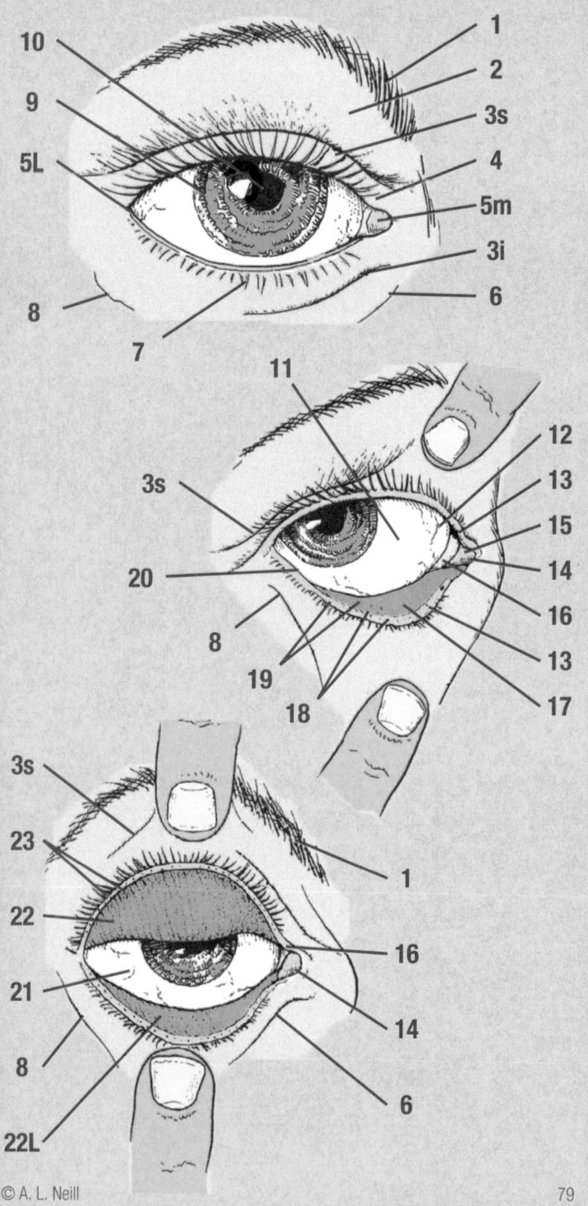
10
9
5L
8
7
1
2
3s
4
5m
3i
6
11
3s
20
8
19
18
12
13
15
14
16
13
17
3s
23
22
21
8
22L
1
16
14
6

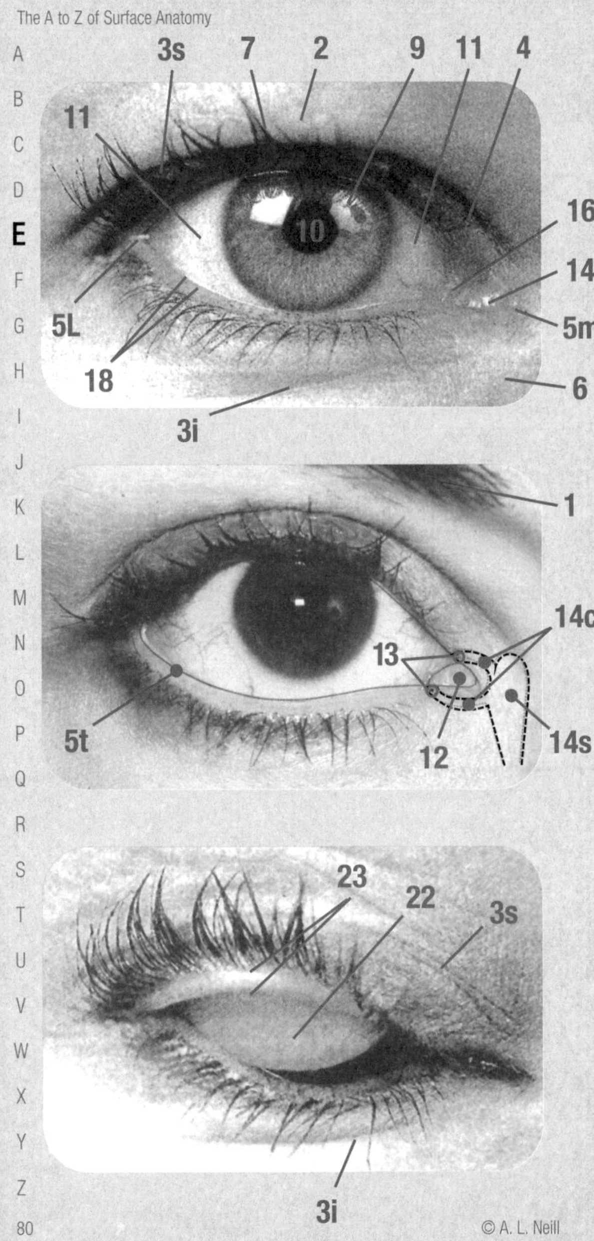
A
B
C
D
E
F
G
H
I
J
K
L
M
N
O
P
Q
R
S
T
U
V
W
X
Y
Z
3s
7
2
9
11
4
11
10
16
14
5L
5m
18
6
3i
1
14c
13
5t
12
14s
23
22
3s
3i

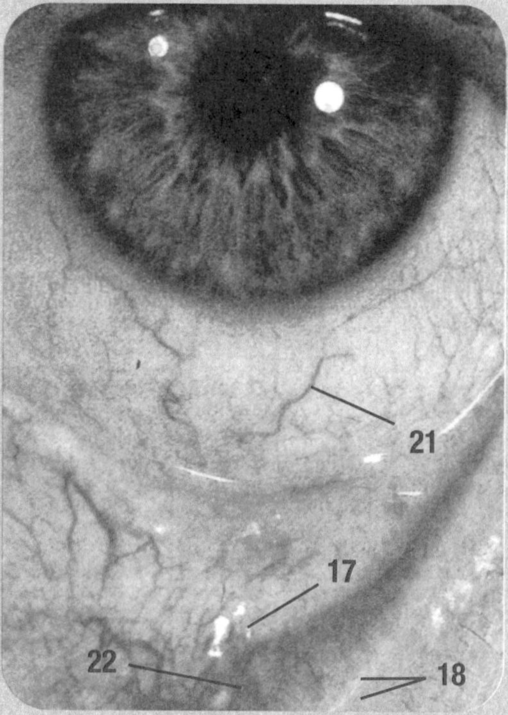

21
17
22
18

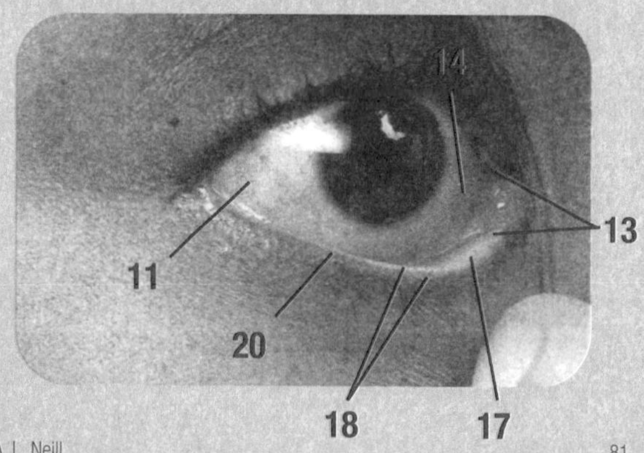

Face – Arteries - major

Anterior

1 Facial artery
2 submental br
3 inferior labial br
4 superior labial br
5 internal nasal br
6 external nasal br
7 angular br
8 Supratrochlear artery
9 Supraorbital artery
(may feel pulse 1 in = 2.5 cm from midline)
10 Superficial temporal artery
11 parietal br
12 frontal br
13 transverse facial br
14 infraorbital br
15 External carotid artery
16 posterior auricular br

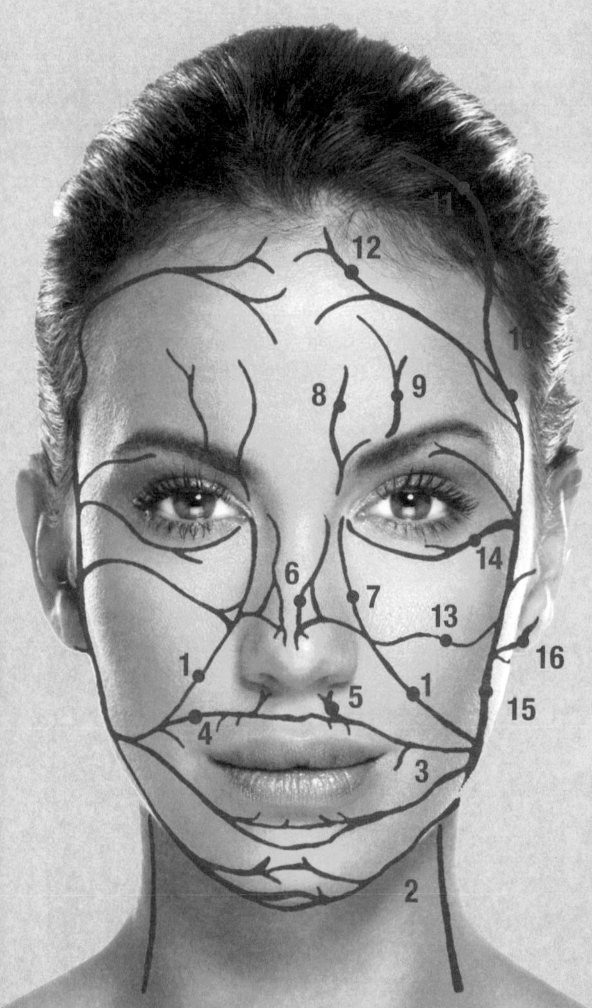
1
2
3
4
5
6
7
8
9
10
11
12
13
14
15
16
1

A B C D E F G H I J K L M N O P Q R S T U V W X Y Z

Face – Arteries - major

Lateral

There are extensive anastomising b/n all the arteries in the face for more detail see the A to Z of the Head and Neck.

1 Facial artery
2 mental br + submental brs
3 inferior labial br
4 superior labial br
5 internal nasal br
6 external nasal br
7 angular br /infraorbital artery
8 Supratrochlear artery
9 Supraorbital artery
(may feel pulse 1 in = 2.5 cm from midline)
10 Superficial temporal artery (may feel pulse)
11 parietal br
12 frontal br
13 transverse facial br
14 infraorbital br
15 External carotid artery
16 posterior auricular br
17 deep transverse facial / maxillary
18 occipital

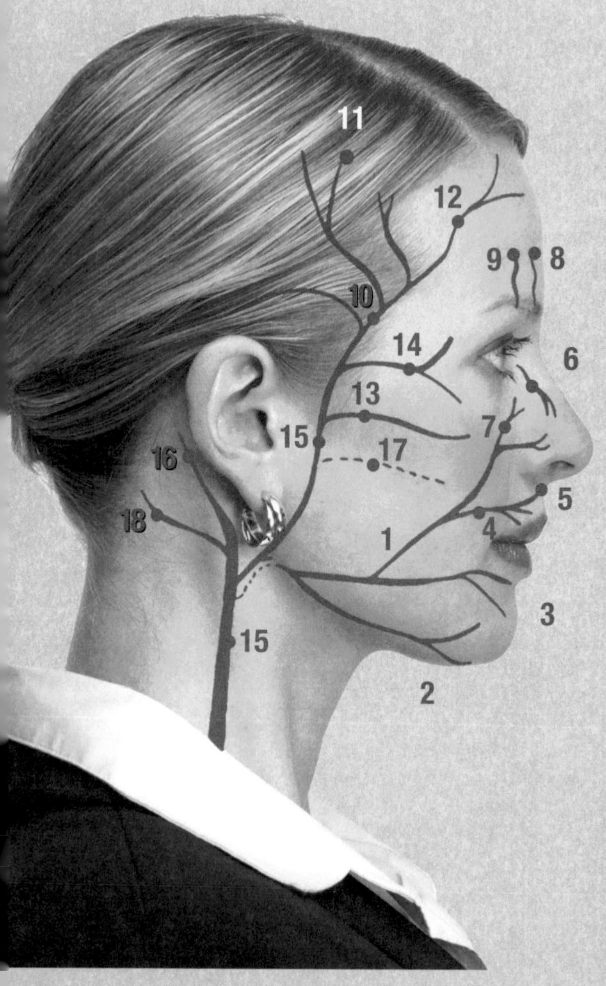
11
12
9
8
10
14
6
13
7
15
17
16
5
18
4
1
3
15
2

Face – Arteries - major brs of the Common Carotid artery

Lateral

1 Common carotid
2 External carotid
3 Internal caotid
4 Superior thyroid
5 Lingual
6 Facial
7 Maxillary
8 Superfical temporal
9 Posterior auricular
10 Occipital

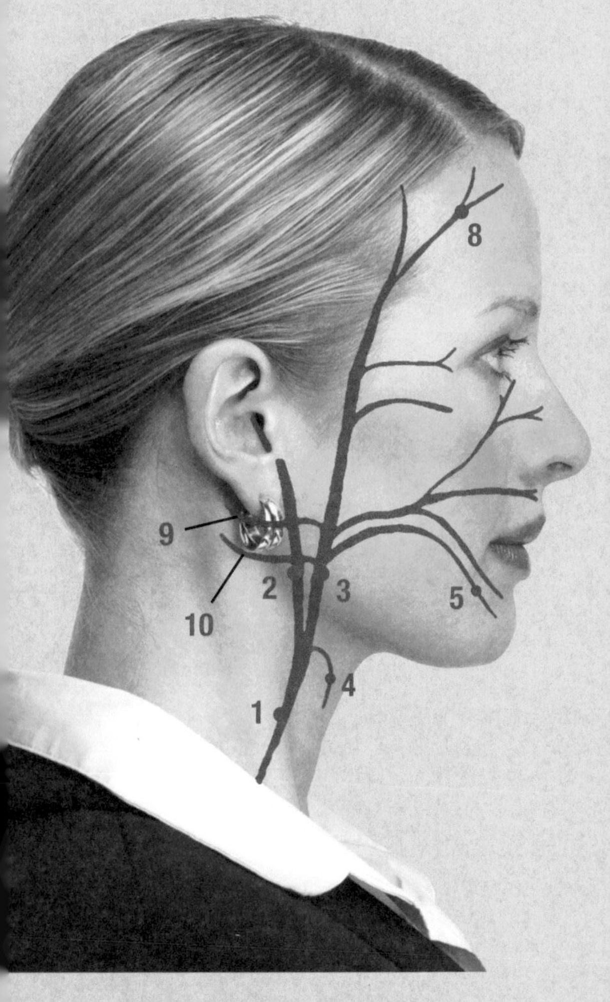
8
9
10
2
3
5
4
1

Face – Bones

Anterior - palpable points - the Brow, Cheek, Chin, Nose

1 Frontal bone
2 superciliary arch
3 suprorbital notch
4 frontozygomatic suture
5 Zygoma
6 mandible a = angle of the jaw
7 mental / chin prominence
7f mental foramen
8 Maxilla
9 infra orbital foramen
10 cheek prominence
11 zygomatic arch
12 Glabella
13 Nasion
14 Nasal bone
15 nasal cartilages
16 orbit

A B C D E **F** G H I J K L M N O P Q R S T U V W X Y Z

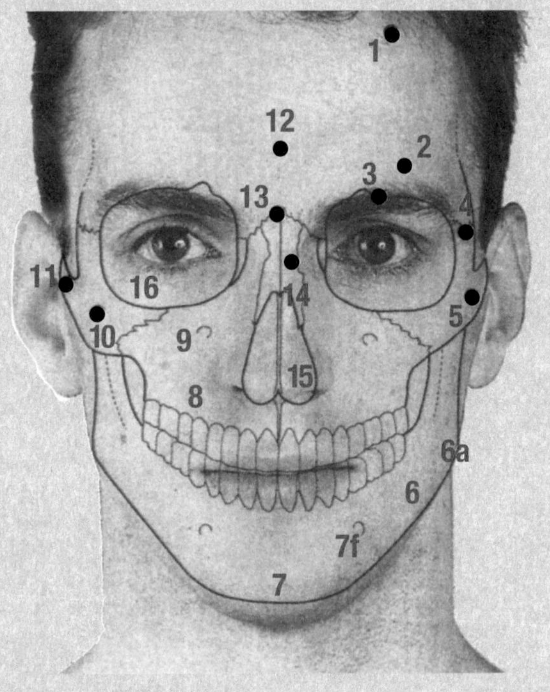
1
12
2
3
13
4
11
16
14
5
10
9
15
8
6a
6
7f
7

A

FACE – Facial N (CN VII)

B

Lateral -

C *The Facial N is responsible for the innervation of most of the facial muscles for more details on innervation of facial structures -*
D ***see the** A to Z of the Head & Neck.*

E The Facial N (cranial N 7) supplies the muscles of the face and some of the back of the head. It emerges just in front of the
F Mastoid process and behind the styloid process - it has 5 major branches coming from 2 major divisions - the upper (7u) and the
G lower (7L).

H

1 Temporal br of the Facial N

I

2 Zygomatic br

J

3 Buccal br

K

4 Mandibular br

L

5 Cervical br

M

6 posterior brs

7 Facial N L = lower division / u = upper division

N

8 Mastoid process

O

9 Styloid process

P

10 Mandible

Q

R

S

T

U

V

W

X

Y

Z

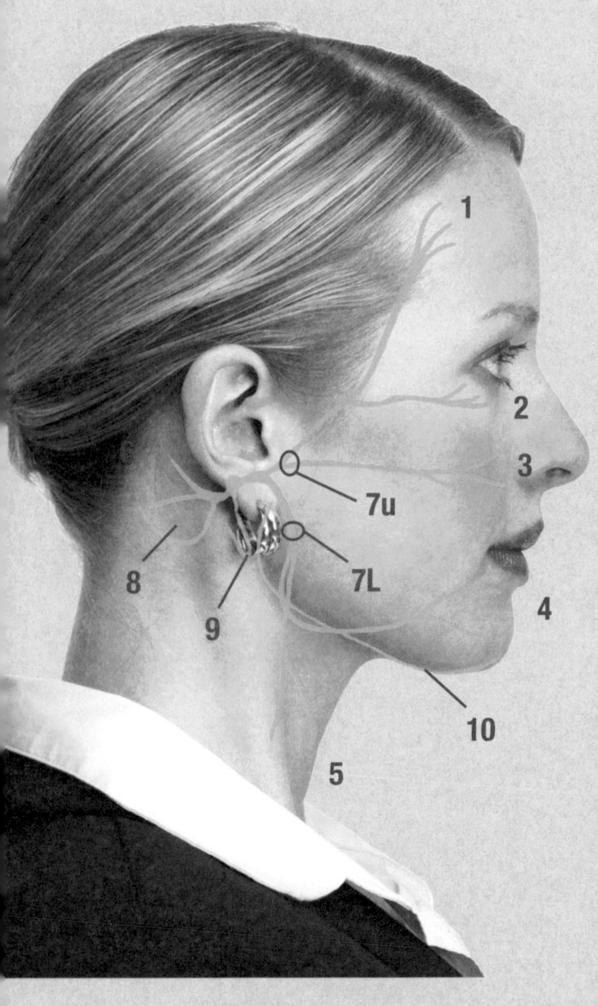
1
2
3
4
5
6
7u
7L
8
9
10

A

FACE – Muscles - major

B

Anterior – only the major surface muscles are demonstrated

C *Approaches through the musculature and major incision sites are also indicated r. For more details on musculature of the face - see the A to Z*
D *of the Head & Neck*

E 1 Frontalis

F 2 Orbicularis Oculi

3 Buccinator

G

4 Orbicularis Oris

H

5 Platysma – partial

I 6 Mentalis

J 7 Depressor Labii Inferioris

K 8 Depressor Anguli Oris

L 9 Buccinator

M 10 Zygomaticus i = Major ii = Minor

11 Levator Labii Superioris

N

12 Corrugator (deep to Frontalis)

O

13 medial orbital incision

P 14 intranasal incision

Q 15 sublabial incision

R

S

T

U

V

W

X

Y

Z

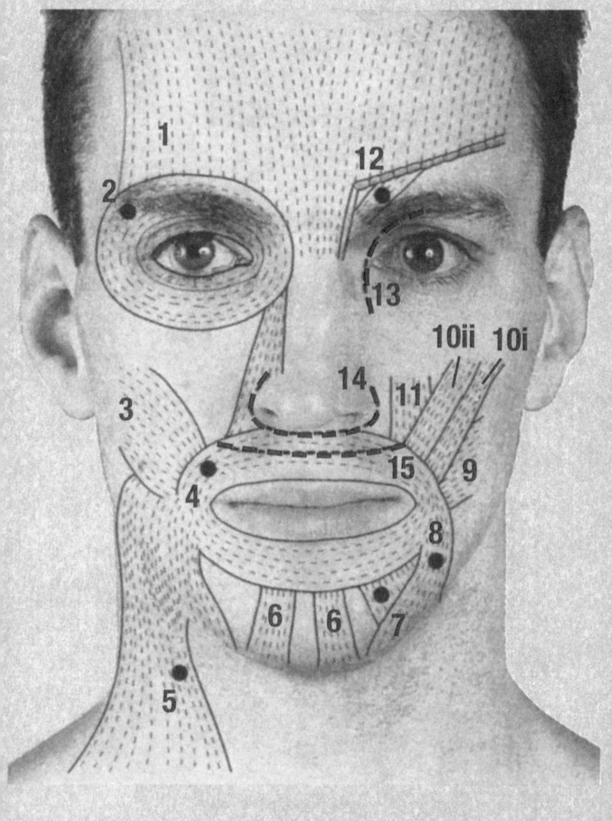
1
2
12
13
10ii
10i
14
11
3
15
9
4
8
6
6
7
5

A B C D E **F** G H I J K L M N O P Q R S T U V W X Y Z

FACE – Veins - major

Anterior - note these vary considerably in individuals

External jugular not demonstrated (see LNs of the Neck) - branches shown in dotted lines.

1 superficial temporal
2 facial
3 retromandibular
4 labial
5 mandibular
6 internal jugular
7 suprasternal jugular venous arch
8 subclavian (R)
9 anterior jugular
10 L brachiocephalic
11 R brachiocephalic

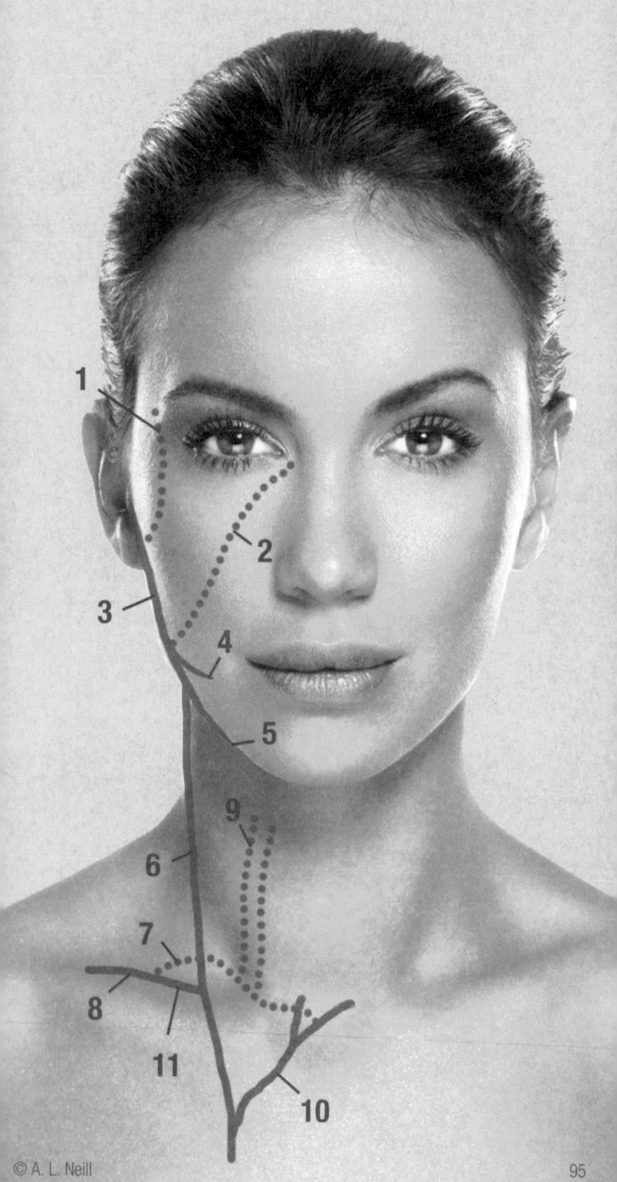
1
2
3
4
5
6
7
8
9
10
11

A B C D E **F** G H I J K L M N O P Q R S T U V W X Y Z

Femoral Triangle – Contents & Borders

The borders of the Femoral triangle are: the inguinal ligament (5) the medial border of Adductor longus (9) Sartorius (10)
The contents are important clinically wrt – LN palpation, access to arterial (2a) and venous blood (3a)

1 Femoral N
2 Femoral artery
3 Femoral vein
4 LN in the femoral canal
5 inguinal ligament
6 femoral canal
7 opening for saphenous vein
8 saphenous vein
9 Adductor longus – medial border
10 Sartorius – medial border

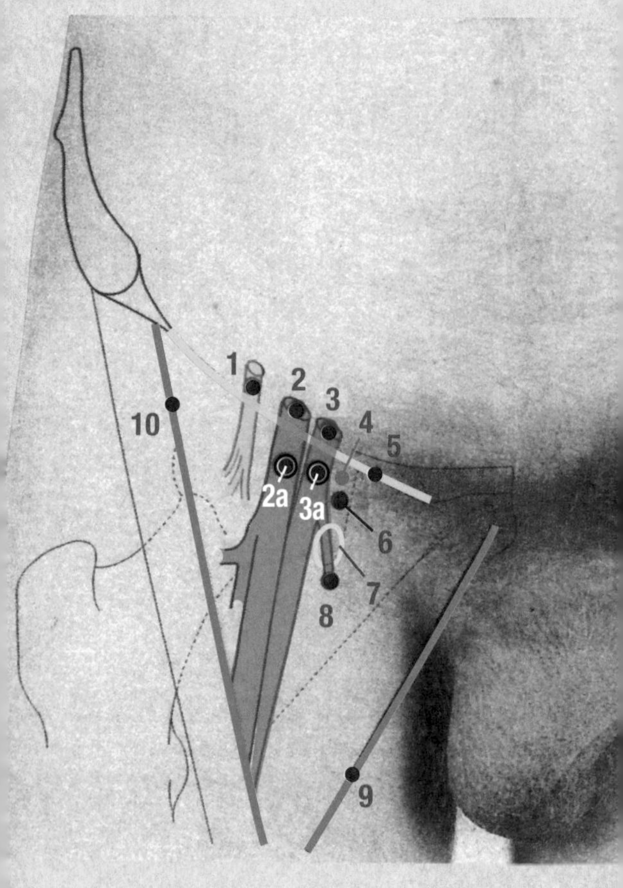
1
2
3
4
5
2a
3a
6
7
8
9
10

Femoral Triangle – Muscles & Bones

These muscles form the floor of the femoral triangle.

1 Sartorius
2 Iliopsoas
3 Pectineus
4 Adductor longus
5 Pubic Symphysis
6 iliac crest
7 iliac tubercle
8 ASIS
9 greater trochanter (Femur)
10 lesser trochanter (Femur)

A B C D E **F** G H I J K L M N O P Q R S T U V W X Y Z

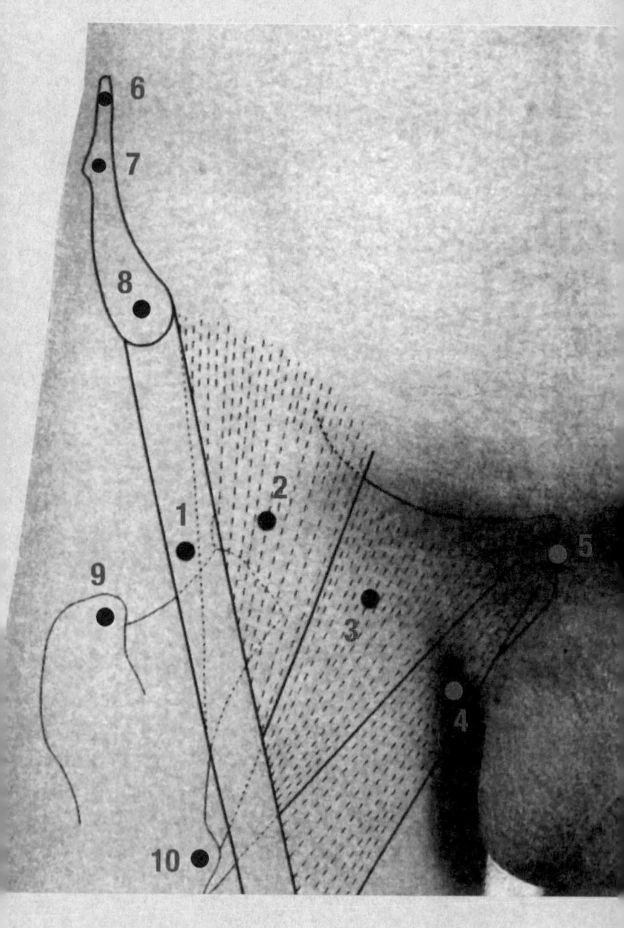
6
7
8
2
1
5
9
3
4
10

Foot – dorsum

Bones

Anterior view -

showing the bones of the foot.

The bones of the foot are arranged in layers as in the hand only with longer MT bones and shorter phalanges.

The only palpable bones of the dorsum of the foot are: the tubercle of the 5th MT (1t), the tubercle of the Navicular (6t) & the malleoli (9.)

1 Ph – all toes have 3 d = distal, m = middle & p = proximal except the Hallux (big toe) which like the Thumb has only 2 t = tubercle of the 5th

2 Tibia

3 MT b = base, h = head & s = shaft

4 Cuniform bones i = intermediate, l = lateral & m = medial

5 Cuboid

6 Navicular t = tubercle

7 Talus

8 Calcaneus

9 Malleoli l = lateral & m = medial

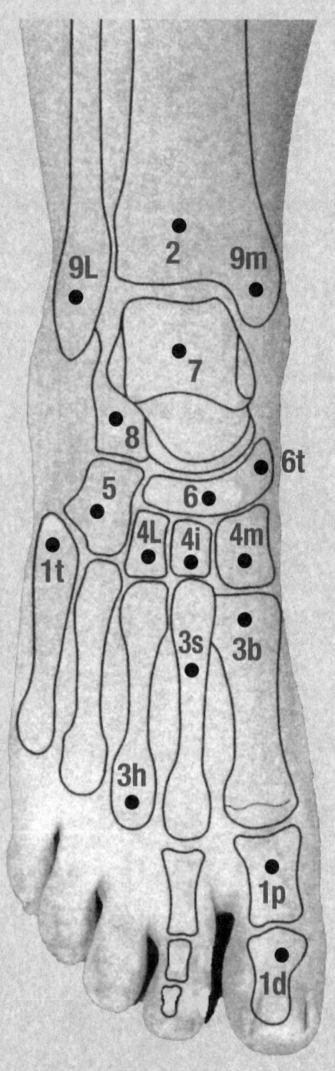
2
9L
9m
7
8
6t
5
6
4L
4i
4m
1t
3s
3b
3h
1p
1d

Foot – dorsum

Tendons

Anterior view -
showing the tendons of the foot.

1 Peroneus tertius
2 Extensor digitorum
b = brevis showing muscle and tendon
L = longus
3 Extensor hallicus longus
4 Tibialis anterior
5 Peronius brevis
6 dorsalis pedis artery
7 1st dorsal MT artery

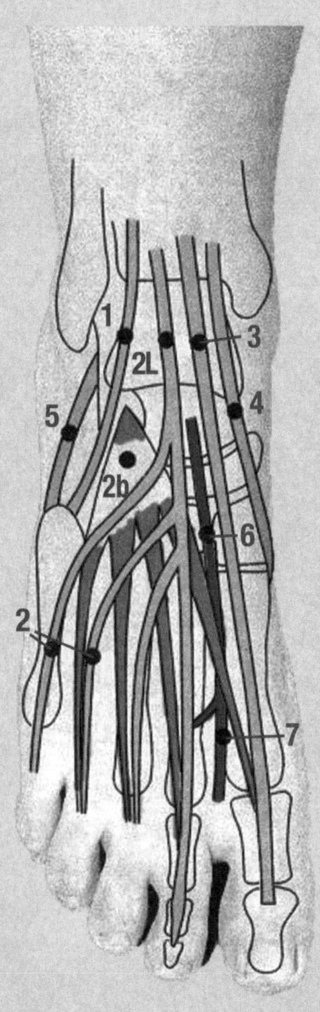
1
2L
3
4
5
2b
6
2
7

Foot – sole Fascia
First layer of muscles

Inferior view

1 superficial transverse metatarsal lig.
2 digital bands – longitudinal extensions of 4 ...
3 transverse bands of 4
4 central aponeurosis

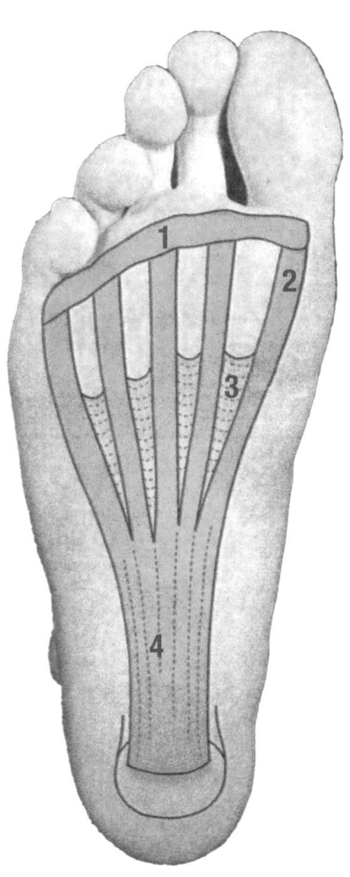

The foot has 4 muscle layers overlaid with a strong protective fascia.

the central aponeurosis (4) is similar to the palmar aponeurosis with extensions (2) to accommodate the extended MTs. A bridging fortified transverse ligament (1) joints all the heads of the MTs to reflect the weight bearing function of the foot

5 abductor digiti minimi

6 flexor digitorum brevis

7 abductor hallicus

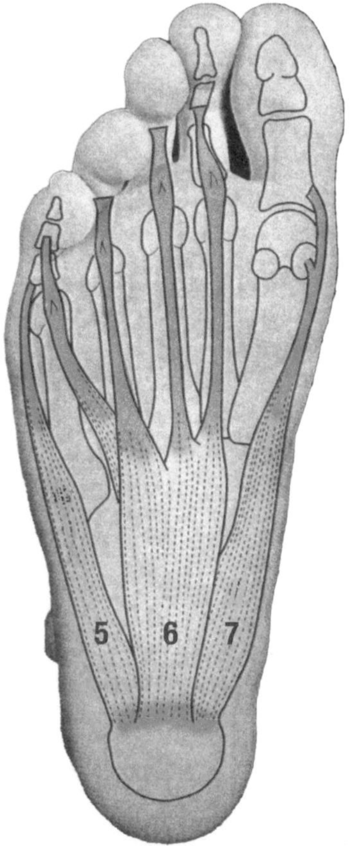

A
B
C
D
E
F
G
H
I
J
K
L
M
N
O
P
Q
R
S
T
U
V
W
X
Y
Z

Foot – sole
2nd & 3rd muscle layers

Inferior view

1 Flexor Hallicus Longus – tendon
2 lumbrical muscles
3 posterior tibial artery and N
L = lateral br
m = medial br
4 Flexor Digitorum Longus – tendons
5 Quadratus Plantae

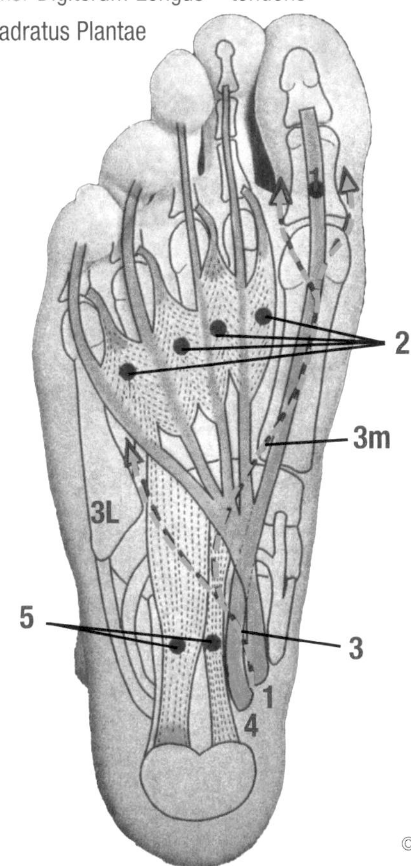

The 2nd layer consists of tendons to muscles which are found in the leg – the long muscles + some of the short muscles (i.e. those completely in the foot itself) – and the BVs and Ns

The 3rd layer contains the equivalent of the thenar (7) & hypothenar (8) muscles which insert into the long plantar lig (9) - technically in the 4th layer.

6 Abductor hallicus

7 Flexor hallicus brevis

8 Flexor digiti minimi brevis

9 plantar lig = spring lig (maintains the medial long arch)

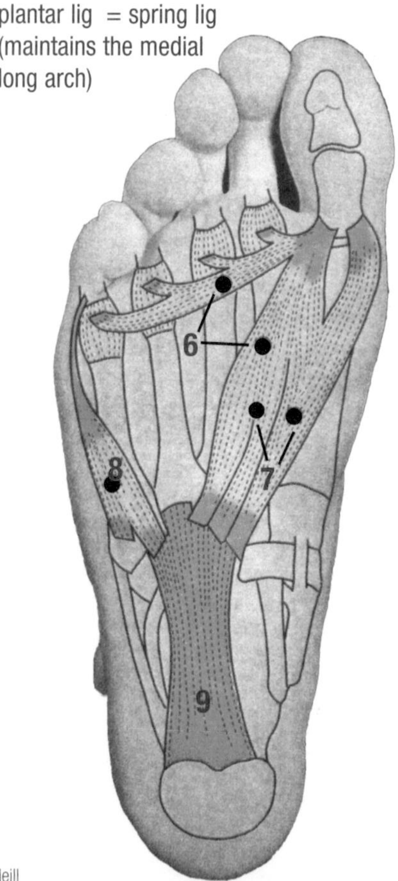

A B C D E **F** G H I J K L M N O P Q R S T U V W X Y Z

Foot – sole
4th muscle layer
dermatomes

Inferior view

1 peroneus lig b = brevis, L = longus
2 Tibialis posterior
3 plantar calcaneo - navicular lig & long plantar lig
4 Plantar interossei

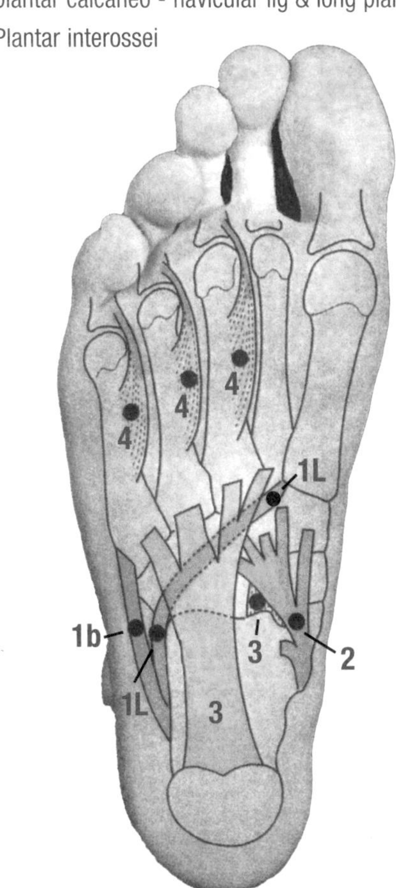

The 4th layer consists of tendons of muscles which are found in the leg and primarily act on the foot and ankle joint. - major lig are found here and deep to this layer which support the arches of the foot along with bony factors

Dermatome distribution of the sole of the foot can be used to test peripheral Ns

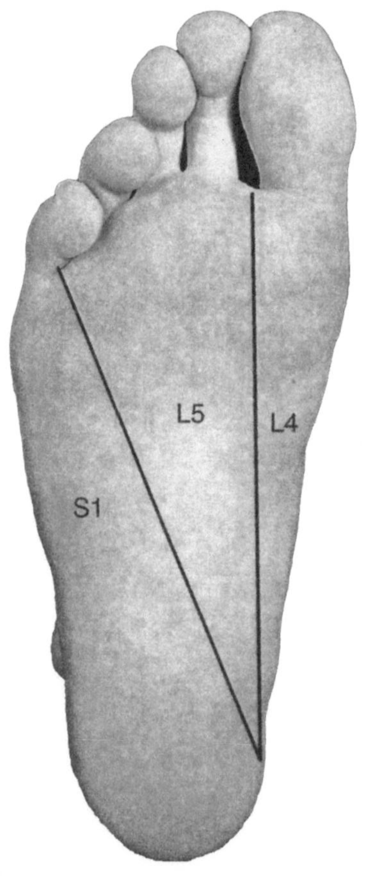

Foot – sole

Bones

Inferior view -

showing the bones of the foot.

The bones of the foot are arranged in layers as in the hand only with longer MT bones and shorter phalanges.

The only palpable bones of the sole are the heads of the MTs (3h) and the posterior aspect of the Calcaneus (8p), the other bones are deep to the short muscles of the foot. The sesamoid bones (2) can be felt over the head of the 1st MT embedded in the short tendons

1 Ph – all toes have 3 d = distal, m = middle & p = proximal except the Hallux (big toe which like the Thumb has only 2)

2 sesamoid bones

3 MT b = base, h = head & s = shaft

4 Cuniform bones
i = intermediate
L = lateral
m = medial

5 Cuboid

6 Navicular

7 Talus

8 Calcaneus p = posterior / palpable aspect

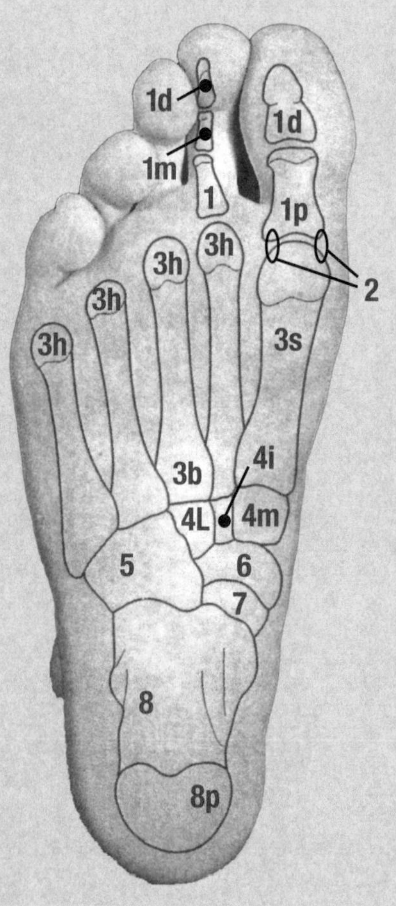
1d
1m
1
1d
1p
3h
3h
3h
3h
3h
2
3s
3b
4i
4L
4m
5
6
7
8
8p

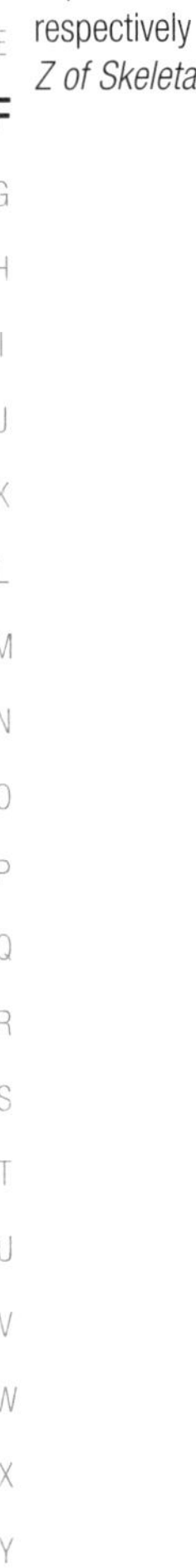

Forearm – Bones Pronation

The forearm in the anatomical position is supinated, it may be pronated by – rotating the lower end of the Radius (3) anteriorly over the Ulna (2)180° while the Humerus (1) remains unmoved this is possible because of the ligaments at the elbow joint and the respectively named supinators and pronator muscles (*see the A to Z of Skeletal muscles* for details).

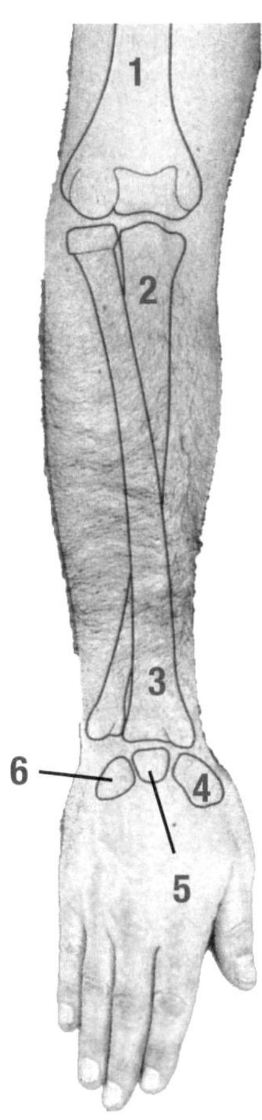

Forearm – Bones Supination

It articulates with the firat layer of carpal – wrist – bones, 4 Scaphoid, 5 Lunate, 6 Triquetral.

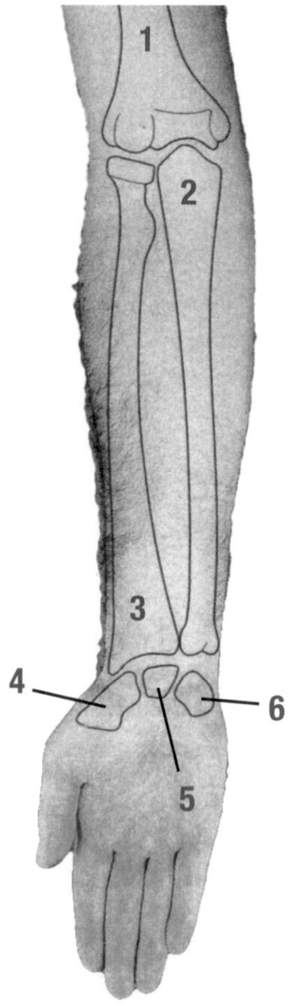

A B C D E F G H I J K L M N O P Q R S T U V W X Y Z

Forearm – Muscles

Anterior (Flexor surface) -

Deep layer of muscles.

The forearm contains the muscle bellies of most finger flexors in 3 layers: deep & 2 superficial layers on the flexor - anterior surface. The tendons of these muscles move under the Flexor Retinaculum (not shown - see Hand) to attach onto the digital phalanges (see the ***A to Z of Skeletal muscles*** for details).

1 Biceps
2 Supinator
3 Flexor Pollicus Longus
4 Pronator Quadratus
5 Flexor Digitorum Profundus

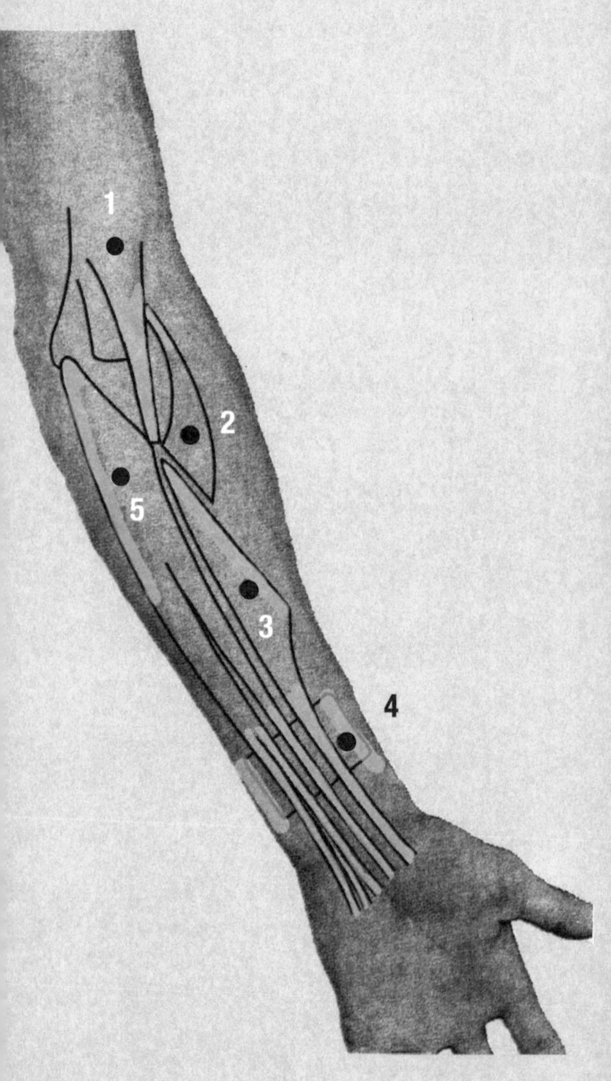
1
2
5
3
4

A
B
C
D
E
F
G
H
I
J
K
L
M
N
O
P
Q
R
S
T
U
V
W
X
Y
Z

Forearm – Muscles

Superficial layers of muscles

The forearm contains the muscle bellies of most finger flexors. The tendons of these muscles move under the Flexor Retinaculum (not shown - see Hand) to attach onto the digital phalanges (see Hand & the *A to Z of Skeletal Muscles* for details).

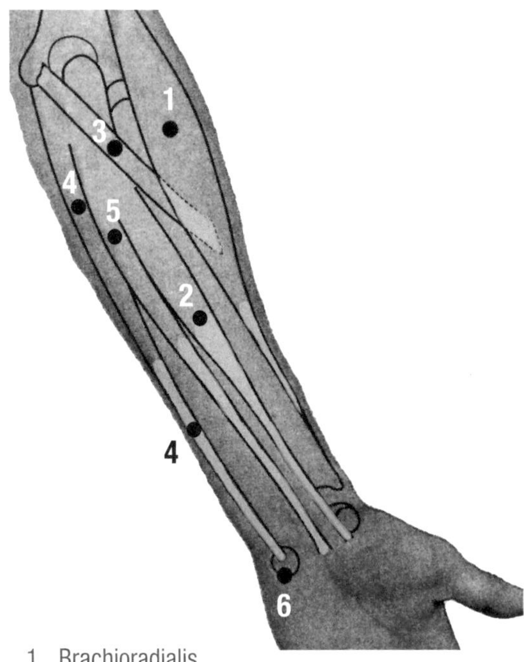

1 Brachioradialis
2 Flexor Carpi Radialis
3 Pronator Teres
4 Flexor Carpi Ulnaris
5 Palmaris Longus
6 Pisiform bone

Forearm – Muscles

Anterior (Flexor surface) -

The Flexor Digitorum Superficialis is the biggest muscle belly in the forearm and lies most superficially – underneath are the rest of the superficial muscles.

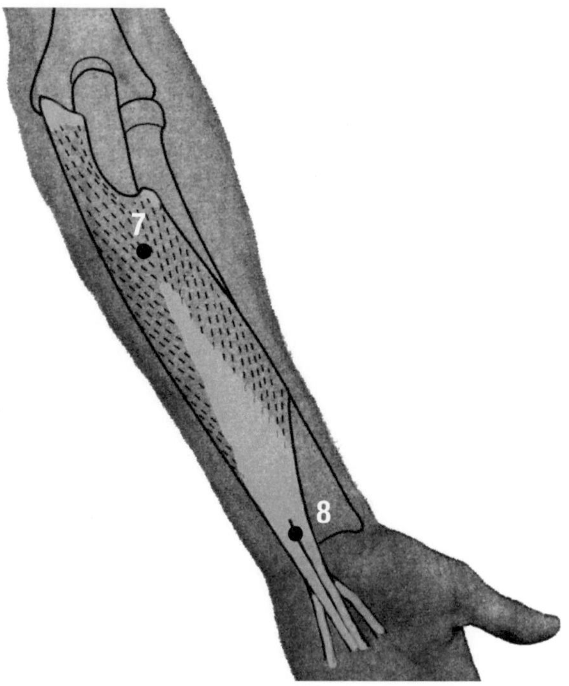

7 Flexor Digitorum Superficialis
8 tendons to the middle and ring figers (lying anterior to the tendons to the index and little fingers)

Forearm – Muscles

Posterior (Extensor surface) - deep layer

The forearm contains the muscle bellies – tendons extend to the phalanges passing under the Extensor Retinaculum (not shown - see Hand).

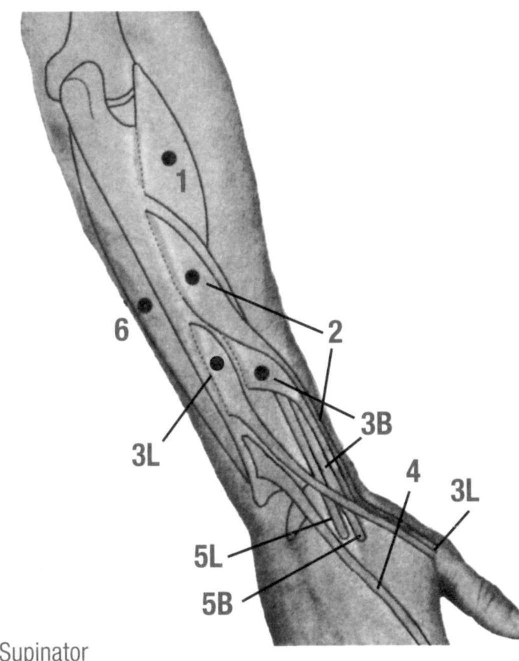

1 Supinator
2 Abductor Pollicus Longus
3B Extensor Pollicus Brevis
3L Extensor Pollicus Longus
4 Extensor Indicis
5B Extensor Carpi Radialis Brevis
5L Extensor Carpi Radialis Longus
6 Flexor Carpi Ulnaris

Forearm – Muscles

Posterior (Extensor surface) - superficial layer

The forearm contains the muscle bellies - tendons extend to the phalanges passing under the Extensor Retinaculum (not shown - see Hand).

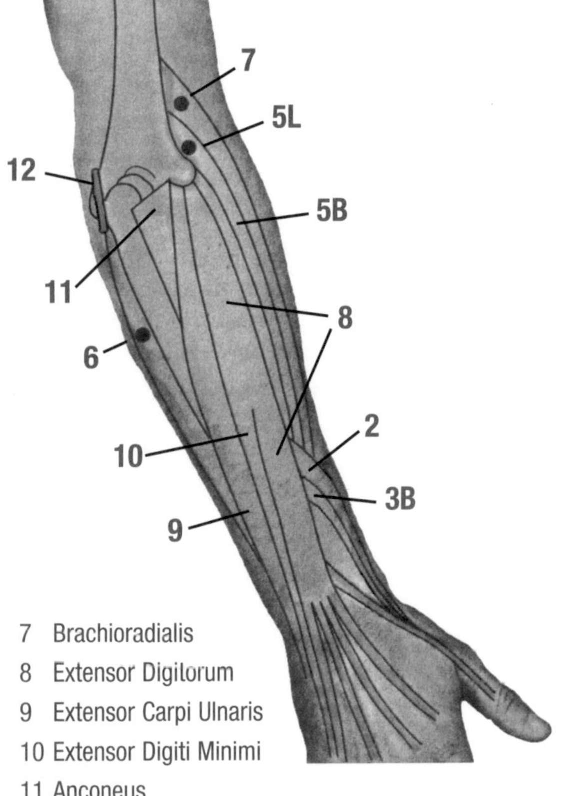

7 Brachioradialis
8 Extensor Digitorum
9 Extensor Carpi Ulnaris
10 Extensor Digiti Minimi
11 Anconeus
12 Ulnar N

A

Genitalia – Female

B

Inferior view -

C

showing the features of the female peroneal area in detail.
Note the Peroneal body is inferior to this.

D

Medium level view

E

1 Mons Pubis

F

2 Labia Majora

G 3 area of hair & pigmentation

H

4 area of smooth delicate skin – less pigmentation

Detailed level view

I

5 Prepuce

J

6 Clitoris – enlarges on stimulation

K

7 Urcthral sphincler & opening

L

8 Labia Minora – edge – engorged on stimulation

M 9 wall of the Labia Minora

N 10 vaginal opening

O 11 fourchette

P Q R S T U V W X Y Z

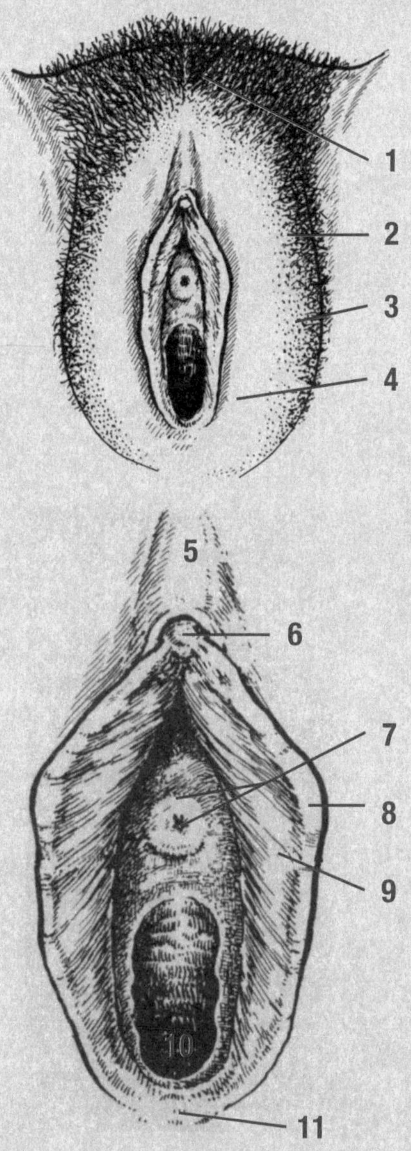
1
2
3
4
5
6
7
8
9
10
11

Gluteal region = Buttocks

Posterior thigh = back of the leg

Bones

1 iliac crest

2 posterior iliac spine i = inferior s = superior

3 sciatic notch g = greater L = lesser

4 L4 spine

5 L5 spine

6 Sacrum

7 femur h = head g = greater trochanter
L = lesser trochanter

8 gluteal tuberosity

9 linea aspera

10 femoral condyle L = lateral m = medial

11 adductor tubercle

12 ischeal tuberosity

13 ischeal spine

14 sacro-iliac joint

15 Coccyx

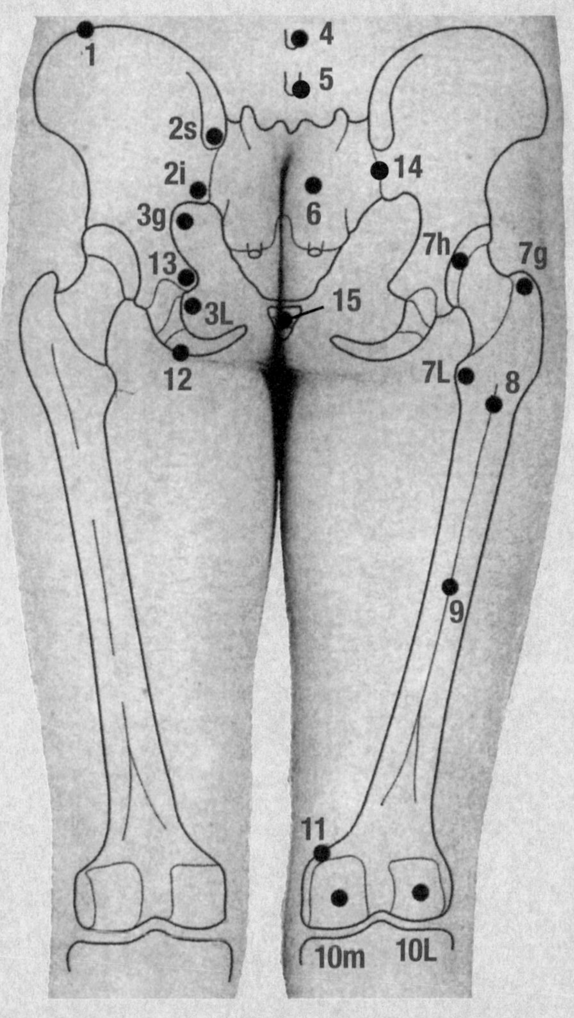
1
4
5
2s
2i
3g
13
3L
12
6
14
7h
7g
15
7L
8
9
11
10m
10L

Gluteal region = Buttocks
Posterior thigh = back of the leg
Muscles + Sciatic N

1 Tensor fascia lata small muscle - long tendon

2 Gluteal muscles
i = Gluteus Maximus
ii = Gluteus Medius
iii = Gluteus Minimus (deepest)

3 PSIS

4 4s - sacrospinous lig 4t – sacrotuberous lig

5 Piriformis

6 Quadratus Femoris m

7 Adductor Magnus m

8 Gracilis m

9 Adductor hiatus

10 Biceps femoris L = long head, s = short head

11 Semitendinous m

12 Semimembranous m

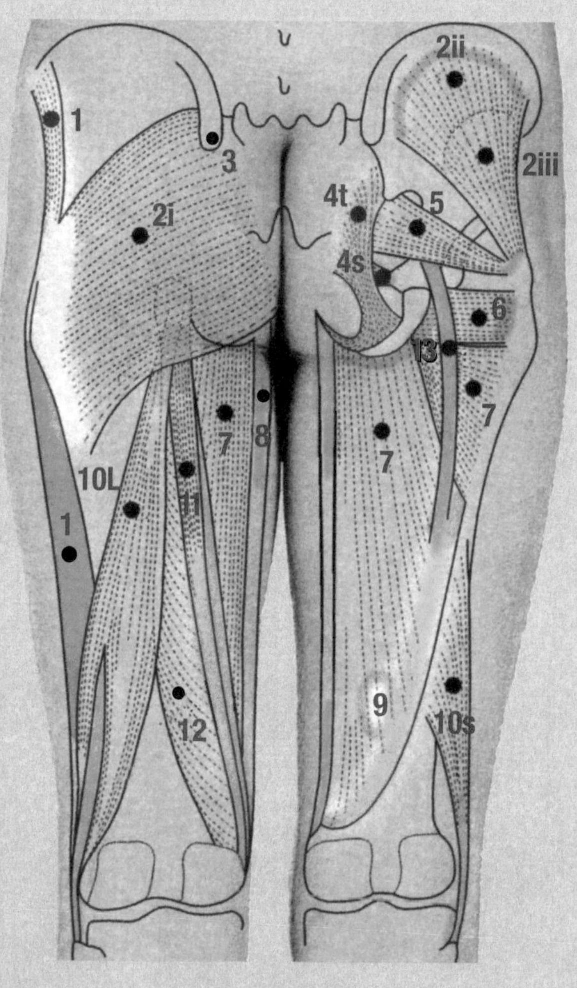
1
2i
3
2ii
2iii
4t
5
4s
6
13
7
8
7
7
10L
11
1
9
10s
12

A B C D E F G H I J K L M N O P Q R S T U V W X Y Z

Hand – Bones
Dorsal surface

1 Ph = Phalanges d = distal, m = middle, p = proximal
2 MC
3 Radius s = styloid process, t = dorsal tubercle
4 Ulna s = styloid process
5 Trapezium
6 Trapezoid

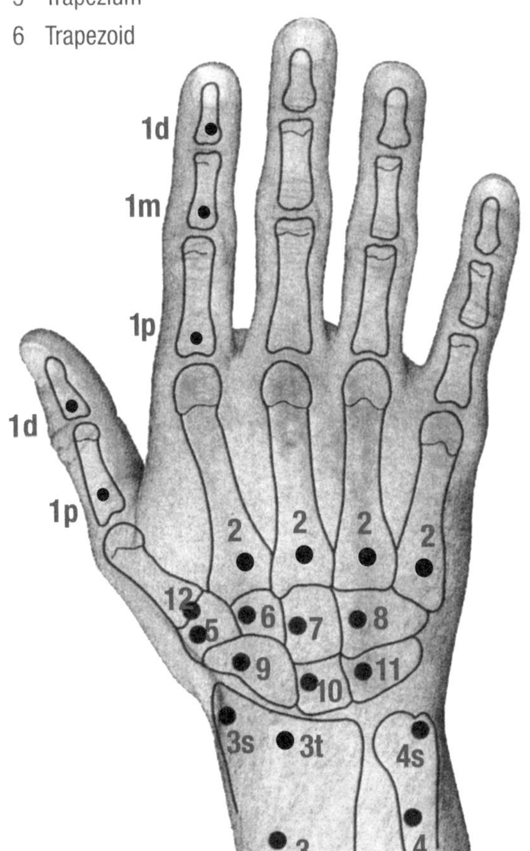

Hand – Bones
Palmar surface

7 Capitate
8 Hamate h = hook of
9 Scaphoid t = tubercle
10 Lunate
11 Triquetral
12 C - MC joint of the thumb
13 Pisiform

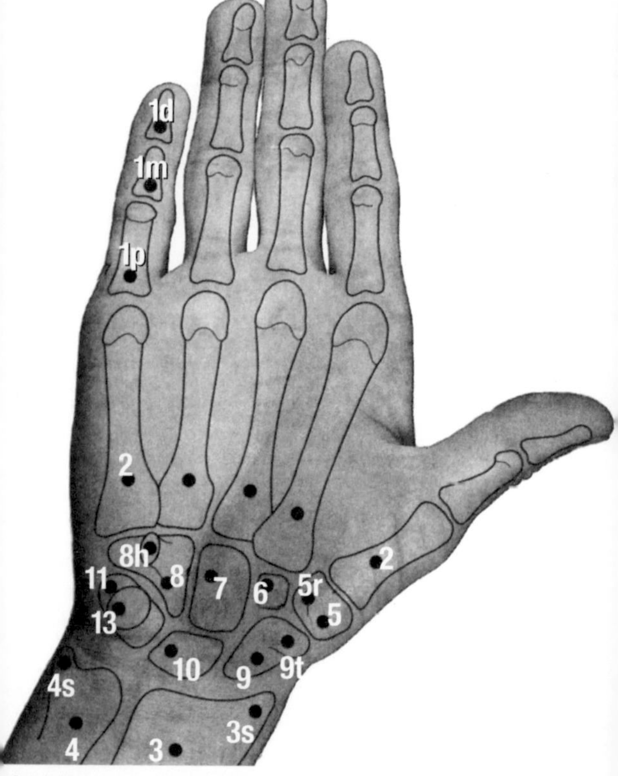

A B C D E F G **H** I J K L M N O P Q R S T U V W X Y Z

Hand – Dorsum

Extensor tendons & synovial sheaths

The hand is highly mobile, hence it must have strong mobile tendinous attachments. To improve mobility these expand to individual synovial sheaths commencing from the base of the fingers.

1 Abductor pollicus longus
2 Extensor pollicus brevis
3 Extensor carpi radialis longus
4 Extensor carpi radialis brevis
5 Extensor pollicus longus
6 Extensor indicis
7 Extensor digitorum (communicans)
8 Extensor digit minimi
9 Extensor carpi ulnaris – in supination / shown more laterally as in pronation
10 Extensor retinaculum
11 shared synovial bursa of extensors

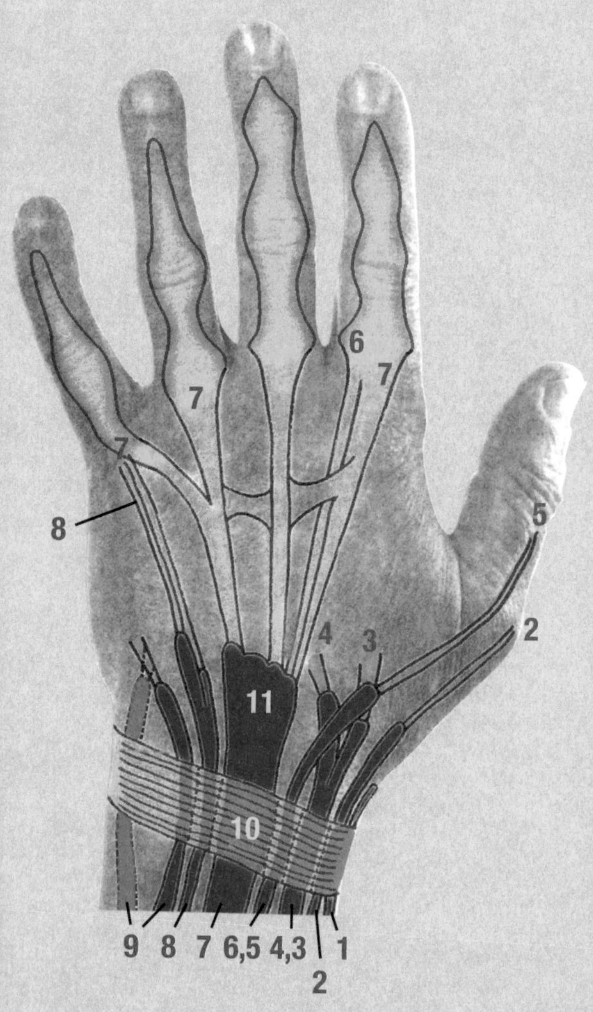

6
7
7
7
8
5
2
4
3
11
10
9
8
7
6,5
4,3
2
1

A B C D E F G **H** I J K L M N O P Q R S T U V W X Y Z

Hand - Palm

Features

The palm has many different features depending upon its function, but several are consistently found in most hands, which include:the 3 primary palmar creases which usually do not intersect (3d, 3p,5) the thenar and hypothenar eminences, the finger and palm pads.

The combining of the 2 transverse creases (3d, 3p) may be referred to as the Simian line and has been found on the palms of several genetic disease states in particular Down's syndrome.

1 digital creases overlying - IP jt d = distal p = proximal

2 proximal digital crease overlying MCP jt

3 transverse palmar creases surface d = distal
p = proximal
b/n the palmar surfaces distal & proximal

4H hypothenar eminence

4T thenar eminence

5 thenar crease = longitudinal crease

6 wrist creases d = distal p = proximal / carpal tunnel

7 tendon of Palmaris longus (inserting into the Flexor Retinaculum) may be absent – note the tendons Flexor Digitorum Superficialis go deep to this

8 proximal pollux crease overlying MCP jt of the thumb

9 digital crease of the thumb overlying IP jt (only one in the thumb)

10 finger pad

11 thumb webbing

12 palmar pad if prominent may lie in b/n sagittal finger creases

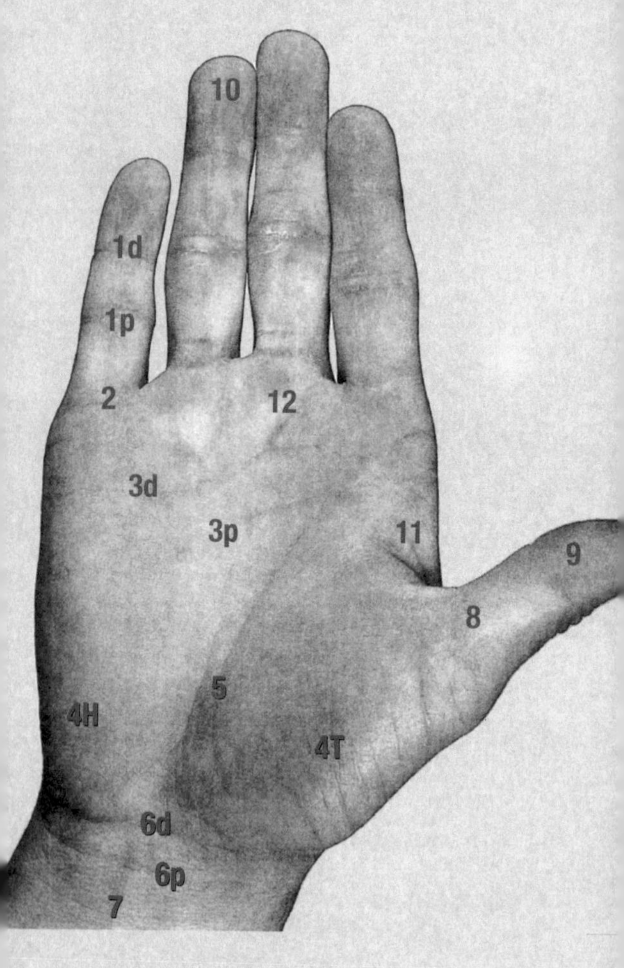
10
1d
1p
2
12
3d
3p
11
9
8
5
4H
4T
6d
6p
7

Hand – Palm

Flexor tendons & synovial sheaths

The palm is highly mobile and designed to grip and hold, hence it must have strong but mobile tendinous attachments. To improve mobility these are housed in individual synovial sheaths, forming bursae, of which only that of the 5th finger is continuous (5) with the palmar synovial bursa (6). With grip changes the tendons would bow if not restrained by strong fibrous bands, (1d, 1p, 2, 7 & 10). These can be identified by their skin tethering, which form part of the palmar features.

1 digital fibrous flexor sheaths d = distal p = proximal (thickened bands of the flexor sheaths)

2 superficial transverse MC ligaments

3 digital synovial sheaths

4 flexor tendons 4p = tendon from FDP#
4s = tendon from FDS

5 digital synovial sheath of digiti minimi, continuous with the...

6 palmar synovial bursa

7 Flexor Retinaculum* (FR)

8 Flexor Pollicus Longus tendon, sheath – note also passes under the FR

9 tendons of FDS and FDP passing together in their fibrous sheath under the FR to the palm

10 thickened fibrous sheath of FPL

11 tendinous attachment of FPL to the distal phalange

 # (note this tendon inserts in the distal phalange - unlike the general rule of deeper muscles attaching under superficial muscles - *see A to Z of Skeletal muscles**)*

** site of carpal tunnel syndrome - this Retinaculum is more distal than the ER*

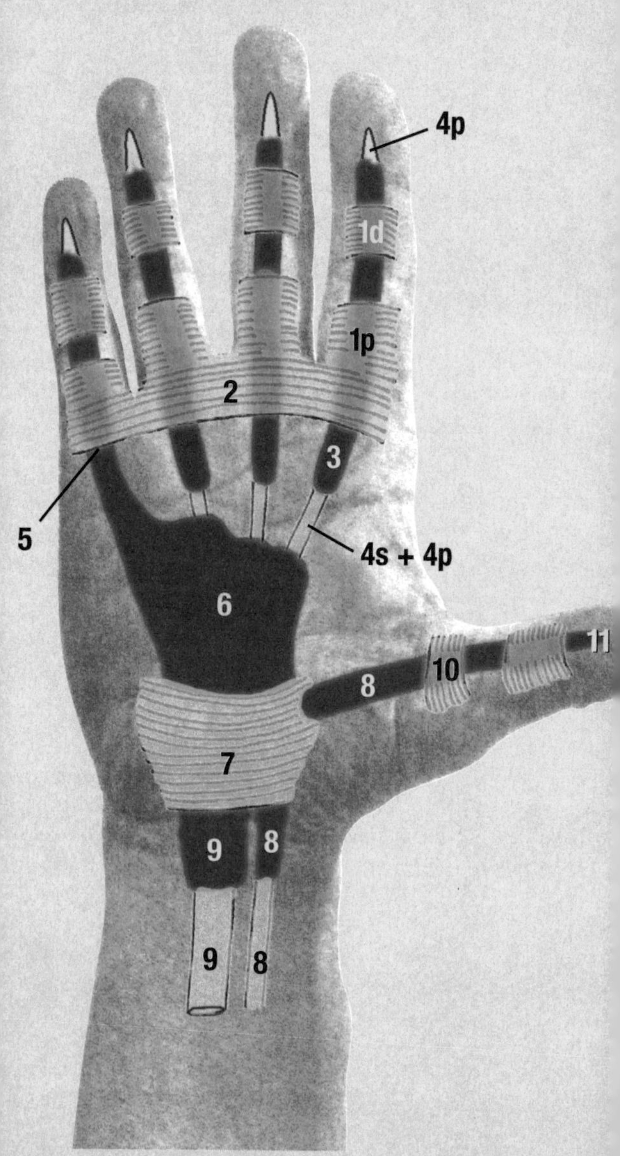
4p
1d
1p
2
3
5
4s + 4p
6
11
10
8
7
9
8
9
8

A B C D E F G **H** I J K L M N O P Q R S T U V W X Y Z

Hand – Palm

Flexor Retinaculum + Nerves

Ns. BVs & tendons pass under the FR, which is an inflexible tendinous sheath connecting the carpal bones and forming a tunnel = the Carpel Tunnel - hence any swelling of these structures will cause pain, restrict movement and may result in tissue damage - the Carpal tunnel syndrome.

1 recurrent br of the Median N
2 ridge of Trapezium
3 Scaphoid tubercle
4 Median N
5 Ulnar N
6 Piciform bone
7 hook of Hamate
8 flexor retinaculum FR

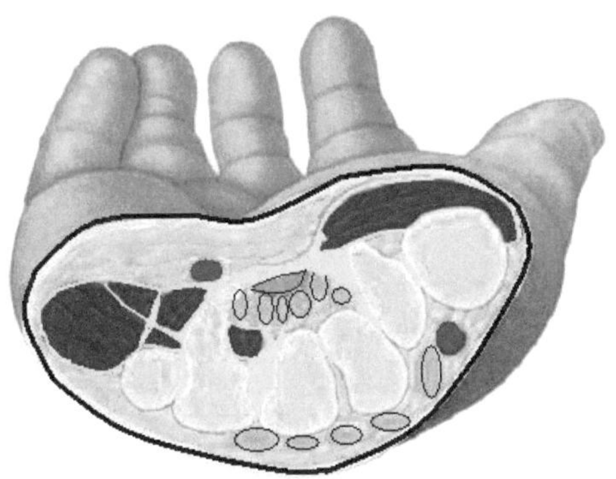

Note the trapping of tendons and Ns under the strong inflexible FR - any swelling as in repeditive injuries will cause pain and loss of function to the thumb, index and middle fingers relived by dividing the FR

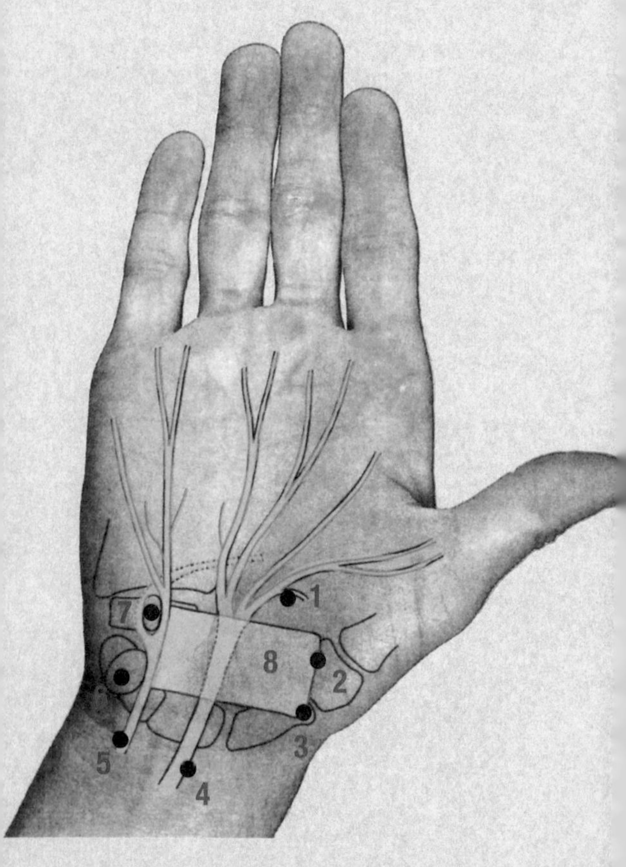
1
2
3
4
5
7
8

Hand
Palmar surface
Thenar + Hypothenar eminences

The bulk of the lateral swelling on the palm is the thenar eminence & made up of the short muscles of the thumb supplied by the median N's recurrent br exiting from the Carpal tunnel (note a test of the median N is to test the power of the thenar eminence) - the medial swelling = the hypothenar eminence (supplied by the ulnar N)

1 Abductor digiti minimi
2 Flexor digiti minimi
3 Opponens digiti minimi

1 + 2 +3 = hypothenar eminence

4 Adductor pollicis o = oblique head t = transverse head
5 Flexor pollicis brevis
6 Opponens pollicis
7 Abductor pollicis brevis

4 + 5 + 6 + 7 = thenar eminence

8 palmar aponeurosis
9 FR

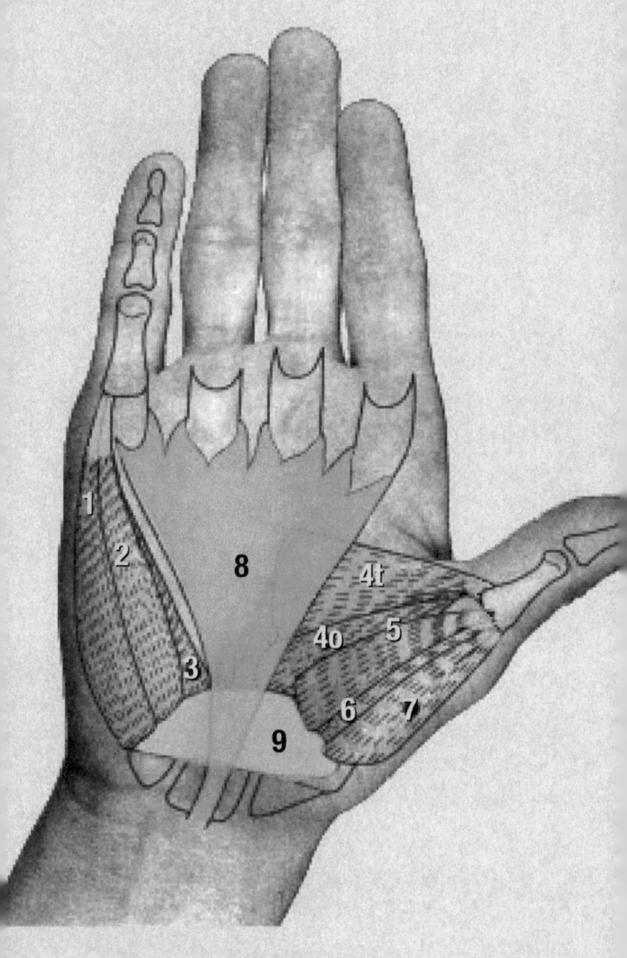
1
2
3
8
4t
4o
5
6
7
9

Heart

Anterior projection of the heart chambers on the chest wall.

1 L common carotid artery
2 aortic arch
3 R brachiocephalic trunk
4 pulmonary artery
5 L auricle
6 L ventricle
7 heart apex
8 R ventricle
9 IVC
10 RA
11 SVC

A B C D E F G **H** I J K L M N O P Q R S T U V W X Y Z

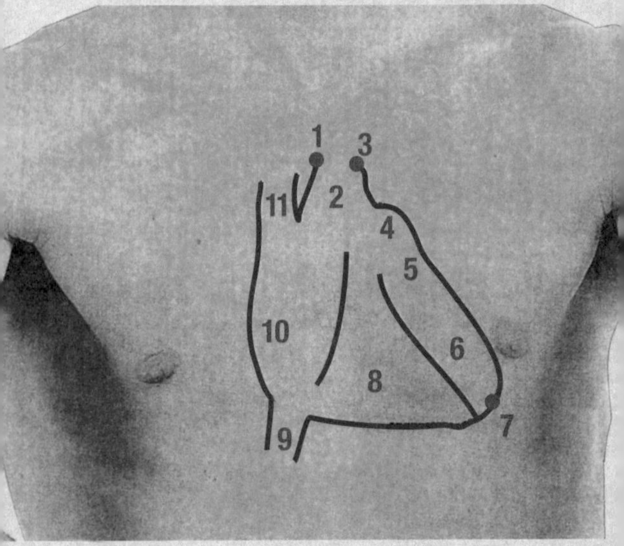

unseen

A B C D E F G **H** I J K L M N O P Q R S **T** U V W X Y Z

Hip – Thigh

Muscle

Lateral view of musculature – deep layers.

1 Iliopsoas
2 ASIS (palpable – ant. & superior to 9)
3 Iliac crest
4 Gluteus Minimus
5 Piriformis
6 PSIS
7 Sacrospinous lig
8 Sacrotuberus lig
9 Greater trochanter (palpable on the lateral side)
10 Vastus Intermedius
11 Body of Pubis bone

The Right angled triangle of 2-9 = Bryant's triangle

If 9 (the greater trochanter) is higher and more anterior on the affected side it is probably due to a # neck of Femur (# hip)

Lateral view of musculature - superficial layers.

12 Gluteus Medius
13 Gluteus Maximus
14 Long Head of Biceps Femoris
15 Semitendinous
16 Vastus Lateralis
17 Rectus Femoris
18 Sartorius

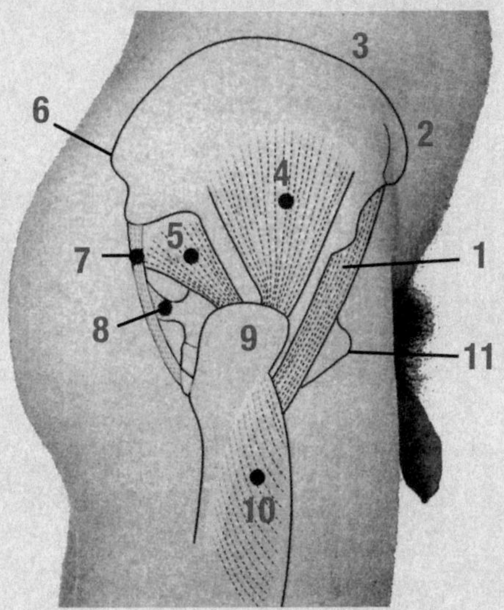

3
6
2
4
5
7
1
8
9
11
10

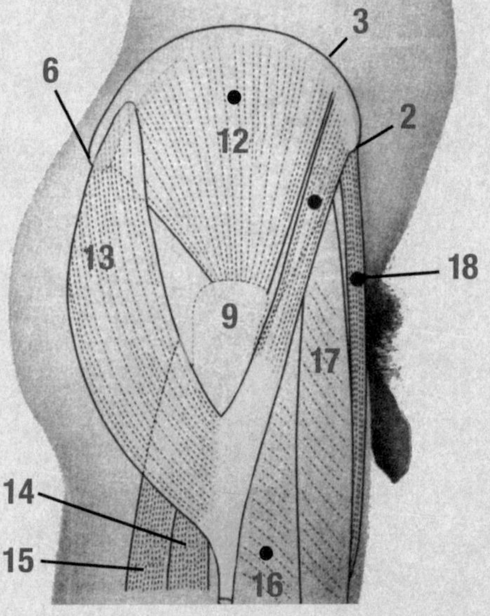

3
6
2
12
18
13
9
17
14
15
16

Inguinal region
Lymph Nodes

Anterior view - showing position of the superficial LNs

Deep inguinal nodes cannot be palpated but communicate with these LNs.

These LNs drain the upper leg, anterior abdomen, perineum anus and lie in the groove of the groin - they may b e palpated normally but are painful and enlarged in infections or malignancies involving these areas.

They are easily examined in the standing patient as demonstrated.

**note the LNs are clinical important in that they are often the first sign of cancer in the drained areas.*

A B C D E F G H **I** J K L M N O P Q R S T U V W X Y Z

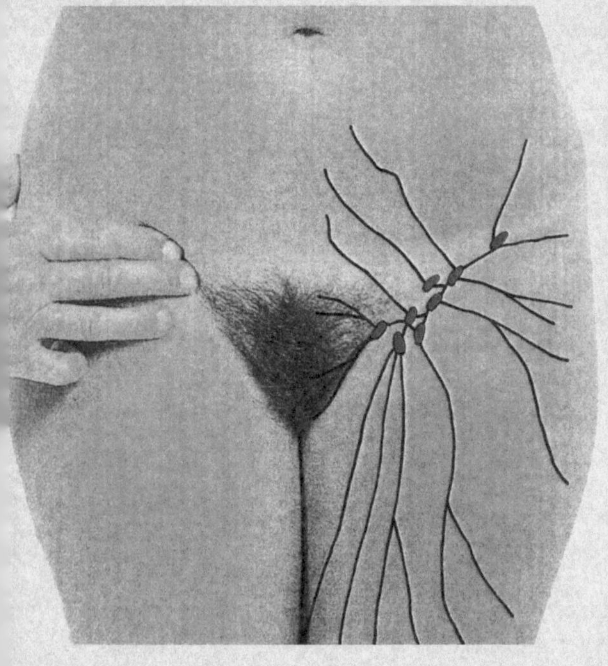

Kidneys – Bladder
Duodenum – Pancreas

Anterior projection of the organs on abdominal wall.

The Bladder, when full, can be palpated above the pelvic rim up to the umbilicus - otherwise in the pelvis.

The Kidneys are adherent to the post. abdo wall - 11cm high - beneath the lower ribs above the iliac crests (supine) - hilae face medially 4-5cm from the midline, as do the ureters before curving behind the bladder. R ky lower than L ky around the transpyloric plane - up to 6cm below it in the upright patient. Posture can affect organ positions by up to 10cm, even if they are adherent to the posterior wall

1 kidneys L & R
2 pancrcas
3 duodenum
4 ureters L & R
5 bladder

A B C D E F G H I J K L M N O P Q R S T U V W X Y Z

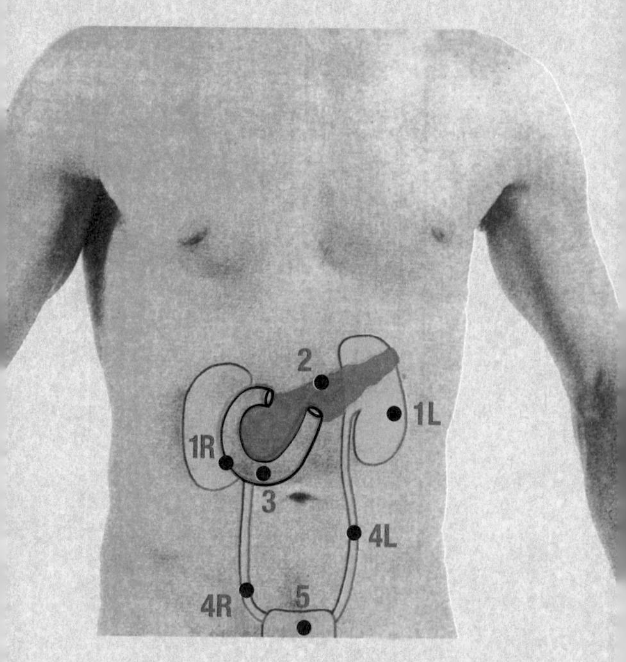
2
1L
1R
3
4L
4R
5

A B C D E F G H I J **K** L M N O P Q R S T U V W X Y Z

Knee – Flexed
Lateral
Medial

The knee is the most unstable joint in the body. It relies extensively on its ligaments and muscles for structural integrity as the bony surfaces are not compatible and provide little or no support.

1 Rectus femoris t = tendon
2 Vastus lateralis 2L / V medialis 2m
3 Biceps femoris t = tendon (note bipennate muscle)
4 Iliotibial tract
5 Patella
6 femoral condyle L = lateral m = medial
7 lateral collateral lig
8 meniscus l = lateral, m = medial
9 common tendon insertion = the patella tendon (bursa behind)
10 tibial condyle l = lateral, m = medial
11 common perineal N
12 head of Fibula
13 Semimembranous
14 Sartorius
15 Gracilis
16 Semitendinous

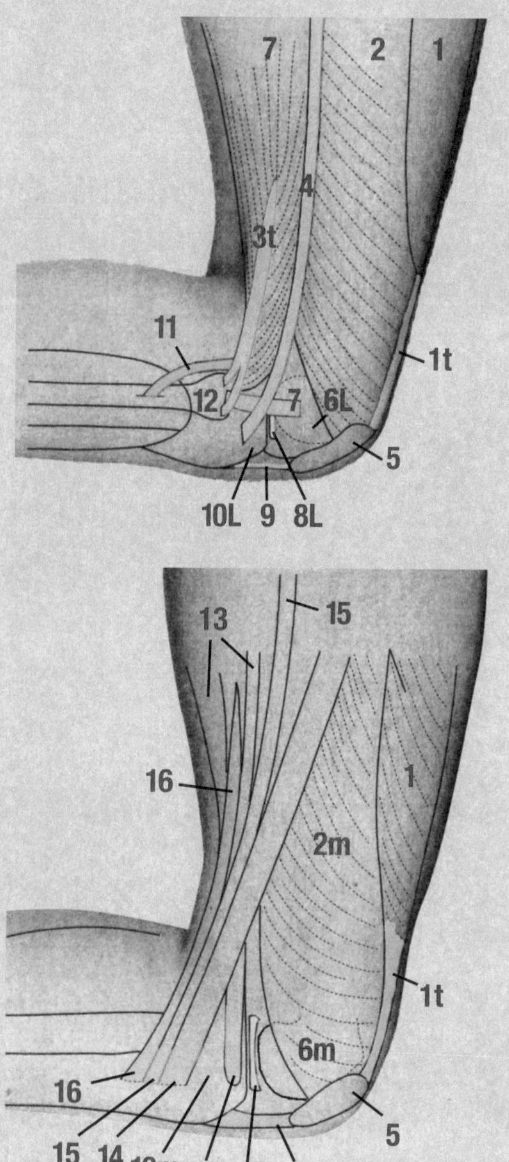
7
2
1
4
3t
11
1t
12
7
6L
5
10L
9
8L
13
15
16
1
2m
1t
6m
16
5
15
14
10m
13
8m
9

Large Intestine

Anterior

Surface projection of the LI showing mesenteries and position in Abdomen.

1 ileum

2 caecum 1-2 ilieocaecal junction

3 ascending colon = Right sided colon

4 hepatic flexure

5 Transverse colon (= Horizontal colon) & mesentery

6 splenic flexure

7 descending colon = Left sided colon

8 Sigmoid colon & mesentery

IS - Interspinous plane

MCL - midclavicular line

TP - transpyloric plane

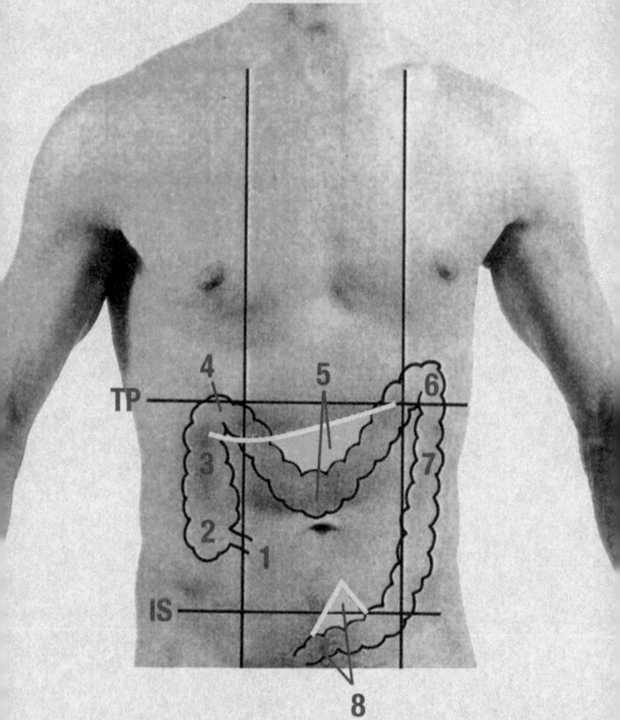

4
5
6
TP
3
7
2
1
IS
8

A B C D E F G H I J K L M N O P Q R S T U V W X Y Z

Lower leg
Muscles

5 views shown –

Anterior, Lateral, Medial, Posterior - deep & superficial.

The knee is the most unstable joint in the body. It relies extensively on its ligaments and muscles for structural integrity as the bony surfaces are not compatible. These muscles & lig attach across the joint from the thigh to the lower leg, in many cases via the Patella.

1 Patella t = tendon
2 Sartorius
3 Tibialis muscles
3a Tibialis anterior / 3p Tibialis posterior
4 Extensor Digitorum Longus EDL
5 Extensor Hallicus Longus EHL
6 Superior ER
7 Dorsalis Pedis Artery- commonly felt pulse main branch - 1st Dorsal MT art.
8 Peroneus Tertius - lig of
9 Gracilis
10 Semitendinous
11 Gastronemius
11t tendon = Tendo Calcaneus = Achilles tendon
12 FR
13 Posterior tibial artery
14 FDL
15 FHL
16 Soleus
17 Iliotibial tract
18 Peroneus Longus & Brevis (L, b)
19 Common perineal N
20 Lateral collateral lig = Tibial collateral lig
21 Medial Collateral lig = Fibular collateral lig
22 Capsule of knee joint
23 Popliteus
24 Flexor Hallicus Longus FHL
25 Biceps femoris t = tendon

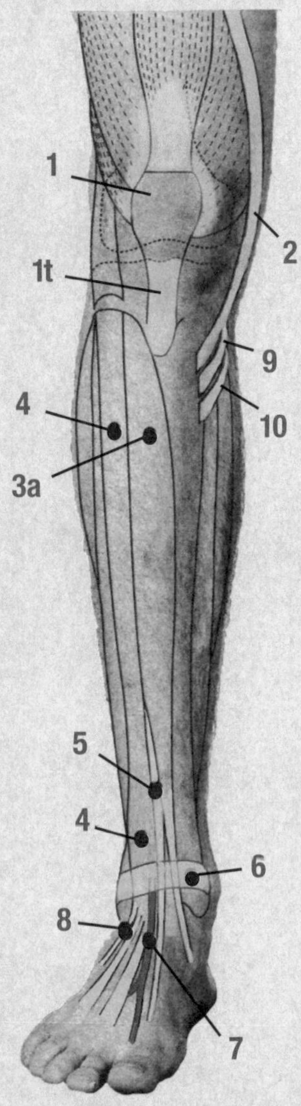
1
2
1t
9
4
10
3a
5
4
6
8
7

Lower leg
Muscles *cont/*

A B C D E F G H I J K **L** M N O P Q R S T U V W X Y Z

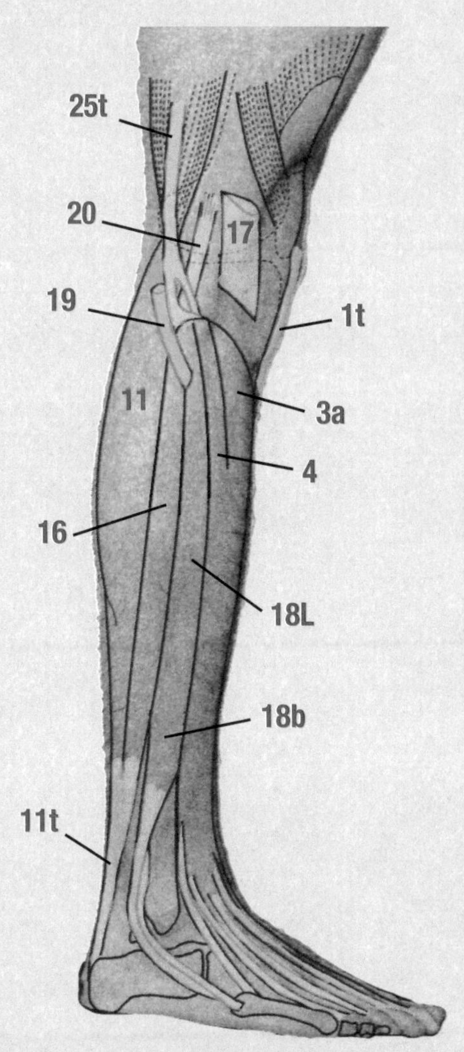

Lower leg
Muscles *cont/*

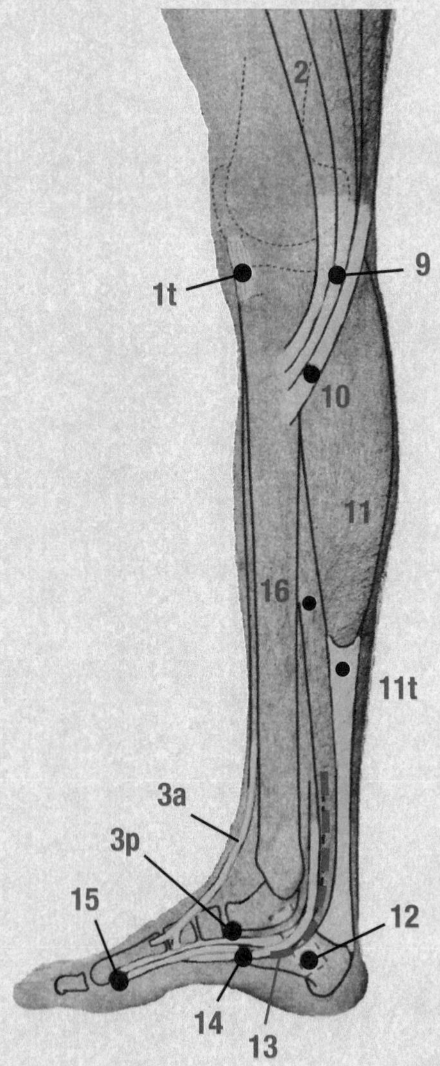

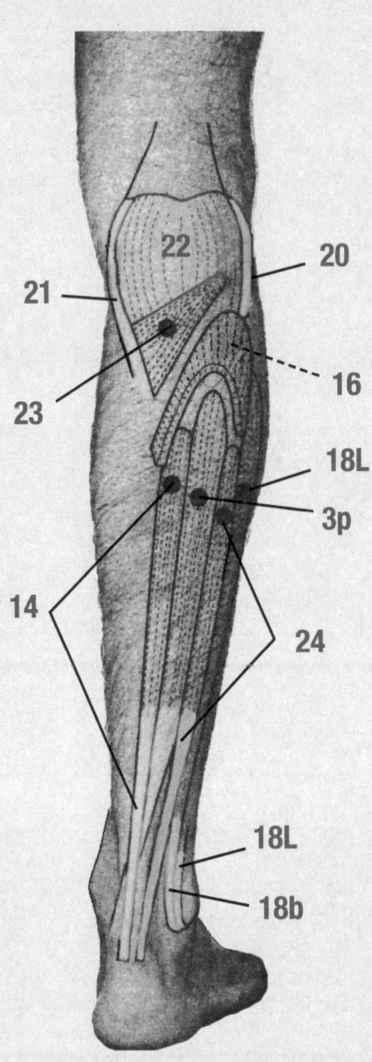
22
20
21
16
23
18L
3p
14
24
18L
18b

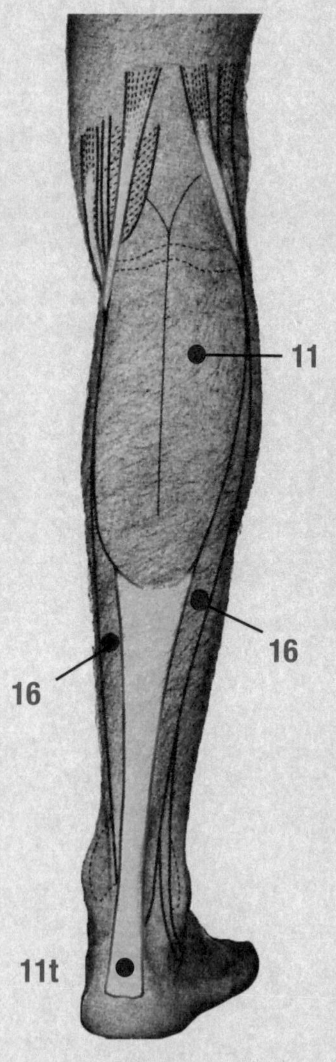
11
16
16
11t

A B C D E F G H I J K **L** M N O P Q R S T U V W X Y Z

Lungs & Pleura

Anterior view with Posterior markings projected through in dotted lines.

The lungs occupy most of the thorax.

They are lined by the pleural sac* - a 2X walled sac separated by fluid to facilitate the respiratory movements. No air can exist b/n these layers.

The visceral pleura adheres to the lungs & fissures – the parietal to the diaphragm, ribs & their muscles. the lungs are smaller and hence the pleural layers meet in areas and do not have lung tissue present in b/n e.g. the costodiaphragmatic recess (3) where fluid can be sampled or drained

2 lobes on the L lung – upper & lower + cardiac notch
3 lobes on the R lung – upper, middle, lower + additional fissure

L left lung - u = upper lobe l = lower lobe

R right lung - u = upper lobe l = lower lobe m = middle lobe

1 outline of parietal pleura

1ai ant. inf. border of parietal pleura

1pi post. inf. border of parietal pleura
a = ant, p = post, i = inferior border note 1-2 cm b/n lungs & pleura

2 outline of lungs / visceral pleura
a = ant, p = post, i = inferior border

3 costo-diaphragmatic recess

4 apical lung 2-3 cm above the Clavicle - parietal pleura = Sibson's fascia

5 cardiac notch - L side 4th ICS lungs + parietal pleural makings

6 oblique fissure - lungs + parietal pleural makings L&R

7 horizontal fissure = transverse fissure - R side only 4th ICS

**note mesothelioma is a cancer arising from the pleura*

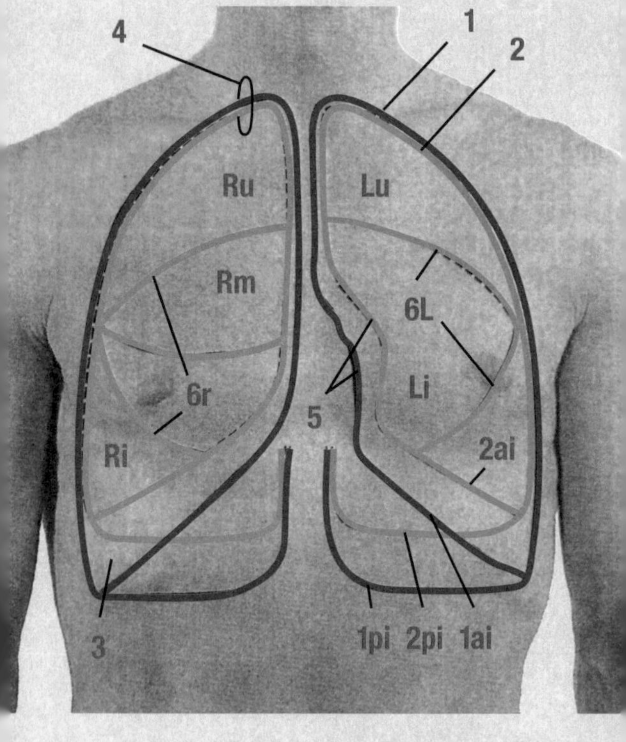
4
1
2
Ru
Lu
Rm
6L
6r
Li
5
Ri
2ai
3
1pi 2pi 1ai

Mouth

Salivary glands

Open mouth -

demonstrating the openings of the salivary glands.

1 opening of the parotid gland
2 2nd molar tooth
3 Hard palate
4 Soft palate
5 Frenulum
6 Root of the tongue
7 openings of the sublingual glands (either side of the frenulum)
7p sublingual papilla
8 Sublingual LNs
9 Sublingual fold (containing the gland and its duct)

A B C D E F G H I J K L **M** N O P Q R S T U V W X Y Z

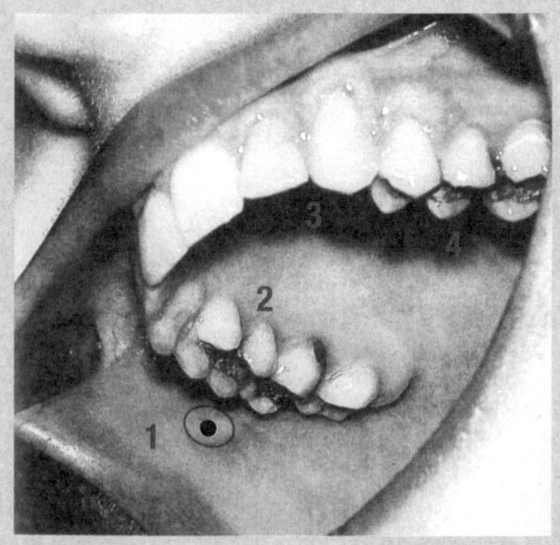
3
4
2
1

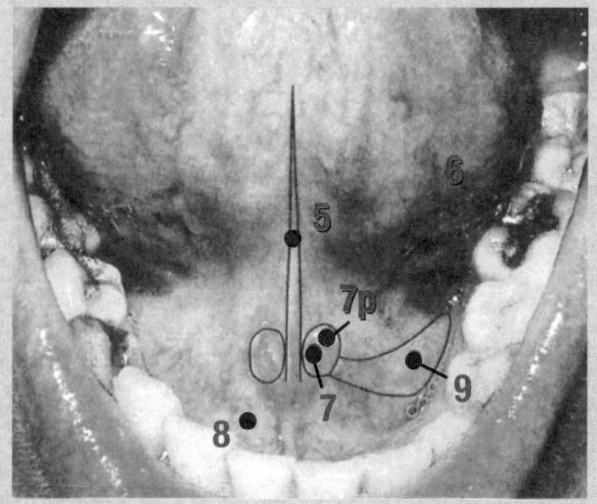
6
5
7p
7
9
8

Mouth

Uvula - Tonsil

Open mouth -

showing the relaxed uvula and tonsil and the raised uvula AHHHHHHHHH. Raised uvula deviates towards the lesion - test for Vagus N (CN X) pharyngeal branch.

1 soft palate

2 Fauces a = anterior arch p = posterior arch

3 circumvalate papillae – b/n anterior 2/3 and posterior 1/3

4 uvula

5 oropharynx

6 tonsilar fossa

7 upper border of palatine tonsil

8 hard palate

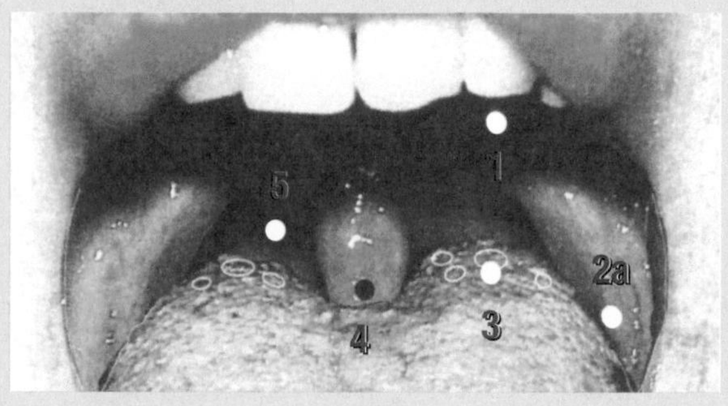
1
5
2a
3
4

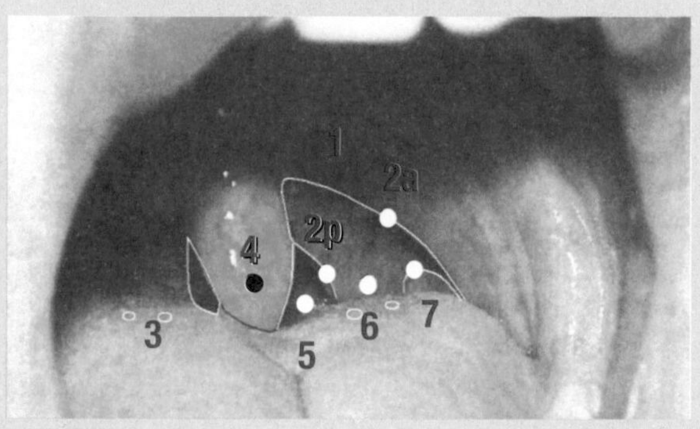
1
2a
2p
4
3
5
6
7

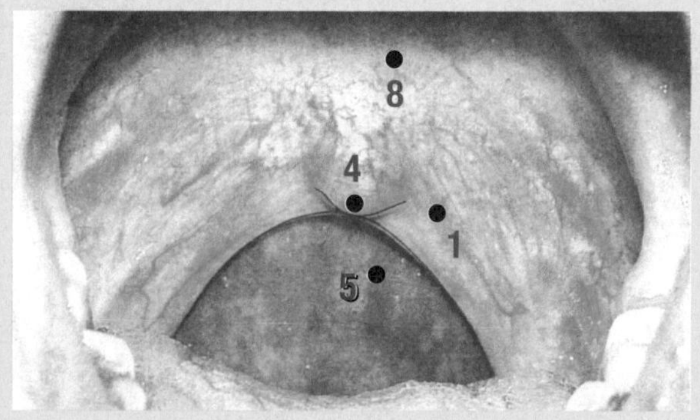
8
4
1
5

Nail – thumb

External view -

of the nail and its components common to all digits.

The nail protects the sensitive finger (toe) bed and is made of hardened protein – keratin. Fingernails grow 0.1mm/day - up to 6X faster than toe nails. Nails grow at a faster rate when damaged.

1 lateral nail groove
2 body of nail = nail plate
3 nail wall
4 lunula = half moon (most prominent on the thumb) region of nail growth and immature nail
5 eponychium = cuticle
6 nail root (in proximal nail groove) is part of nail bed
7 proximal extent of nail bed
8 finger pad
9 free edge of the nail
10 dermis containing nail bed BVs - note more extensive in fingers than toes part of the lateral nail groove
11 nail bed

A B C D E F G H I J K L M **N** O P Q R S T U V W X Y Z

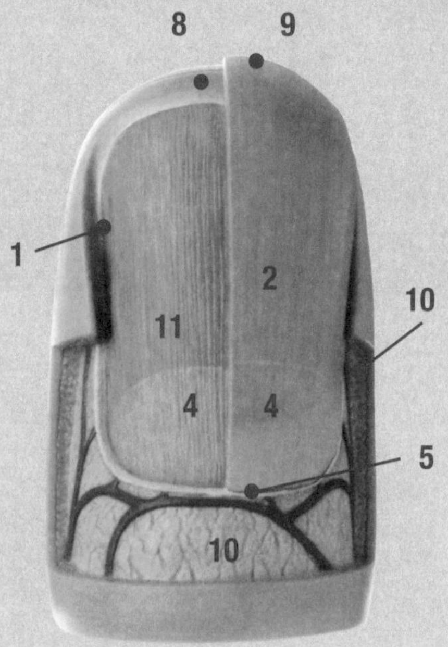
8
9
1
2
10
11
4
4
5
10

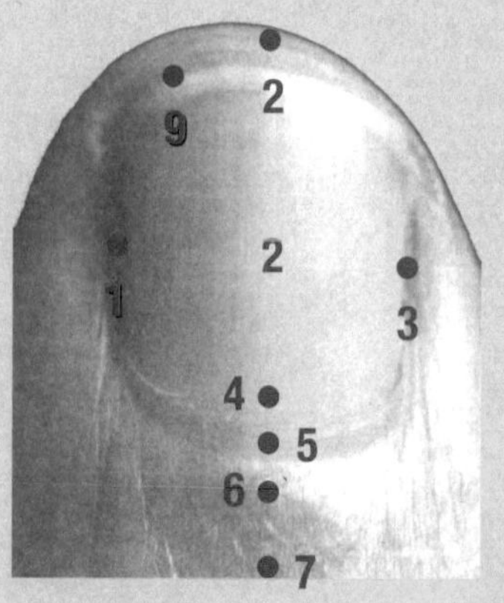
2
9
1
2
3
4
5
6
7

Neck

Anterior view -

showing position of various access points to structures in the neck.

1 Hyoid bone

2 access point to internal jugular vein

3 access point to common carotid artery

4 Cricothyroid puncture site

5 collar incision – for thyroid

6 access point to internal jugular vein b/n the 2 heads of SCM

7 Adam's apple central point – Thyroid cartilage

8 SCM

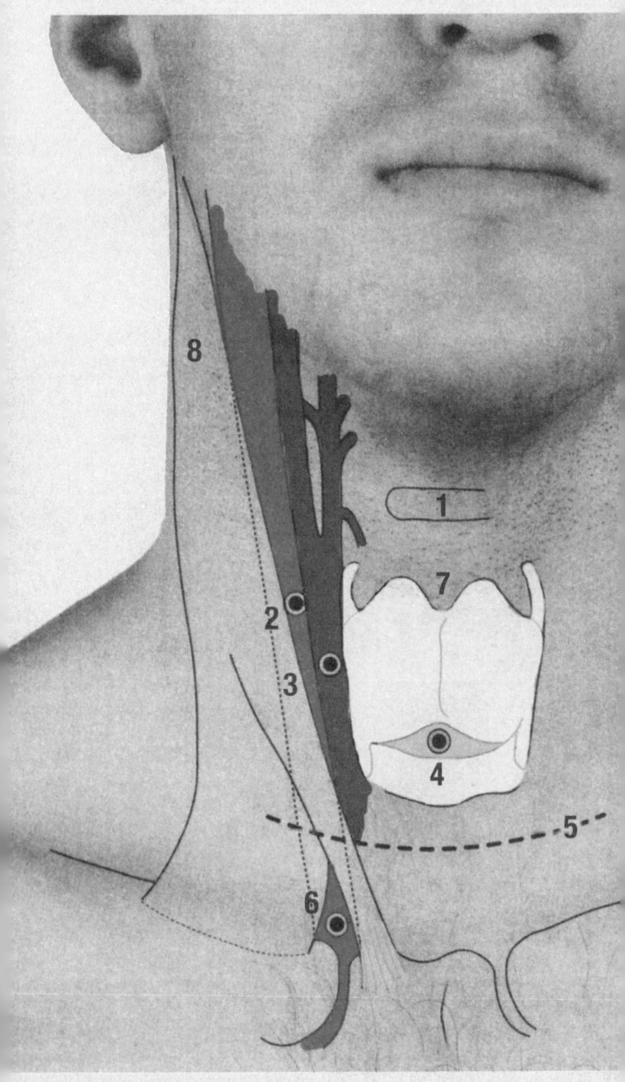
8
1
7
2
3
4
5
6

A B C D E F G H I J K L M **N** O P Q R S T U V W X Y Z

Neck – Lymph Nodes

Lateral view -

showing position of the nodes in the neck.

LNs often surround the major veins & muscle edges –

There is an extensive network of lymphatics connecting these groups, so the order of palpation is not critical

They are the commonest lumps in the neck seen in clinical practice and generally indicate URTI but also cancer or metastases in the region.

1 parotid LNs
2 mental = submental LNs
3 LNs around the anterior jugular vein and larynx
4 LNs around the omohyoid
5 supraclavicular (= Virchow's Nodes*) -
6 LNs around the external jugular vein
7 LNs around the internal jugular vein
8 post-auricular LNs
9 occipital LNs
10 LNs around the digastric
11 submandibular LNs
12 LNs around the internal jugular vein
13 Clavicle
14 Trapezius
15 spine of the Scapula

***note the LNs are clinical important in that they are often the first sign of cancer in the thorax*

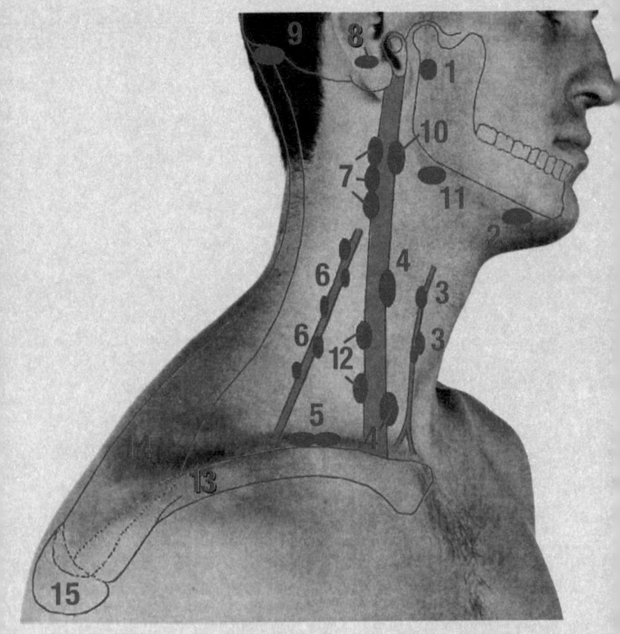
9
8
1
10
7
11
2
6
4
3
6
12
3
5
4
14
13
15

Neck – Submandibular region

Lateral view -

showing position of the submandibular gland in the neck.

The Salivary glands lie in the neck and open into the mouth *– see also mouth.*

1 parotid gland
2 angle of the jaw – Mandible
3 submandibular gland
4 facial artery
5 mylohyoid muscle
6 omohyoid muscle
7 Hyoid bone
8 common carotid artery
9 facial vein
10 surgical approach to the submandibular gland
11 SCM muscle
12 Hypoglossal N = CN XII

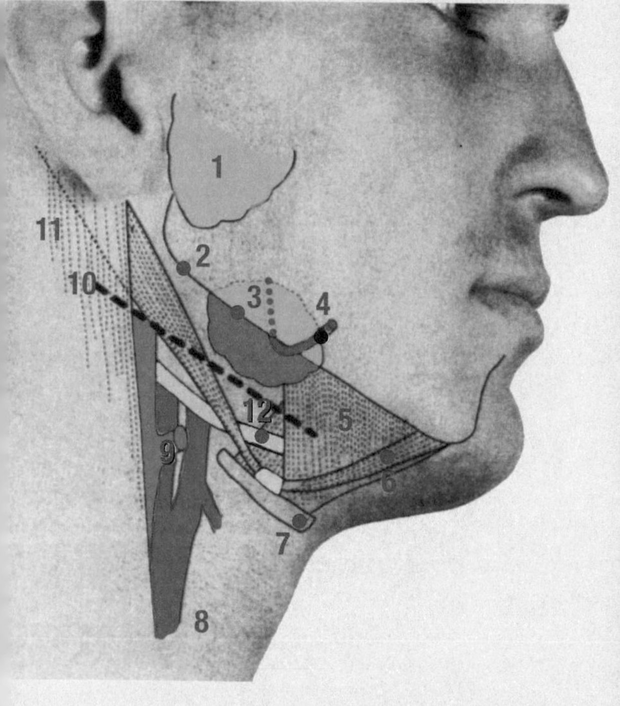
1
2
3
4
5
6
7
8
9
10
11
12

Neck – triangles of the neck

Lateral view -
showing position of various access points to structures in the neck.

1 Anterior triangle of the neck, borders are...
inferior border of the Mandible
midline of the neck
anterior border of SCM

2 Digastric triangle, borders are...
inferior border of the Mandible
anterior border of posterior belly of Digastric
posterior border of anterior belly of Digastric

3 Carotid triangle borders are...
posterior border of Omohyoid
posterior border of posterior belly of Digastric
anterior border of SCM line of the Carotid artery

4 Submental triangle crosses the midline - not shown
borders are ...
anterior borders of anterior bellies of Digastric
symphysis menti
body of the Hyoid

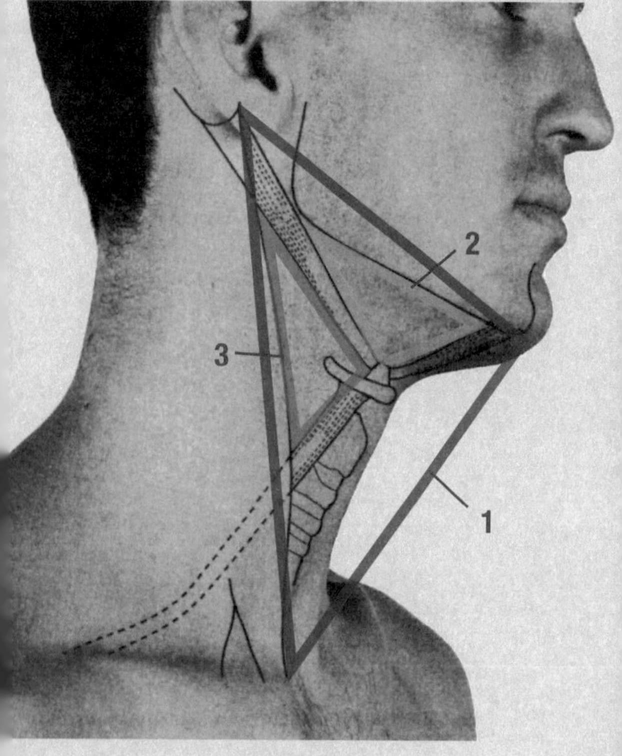
2
3
1

Neck – triangles of the neck

Postero-Lateral view -

showing position of various access points to structures in the neck.

1 Posterior triangle of the neck, borders are...
anterior border of Trapezius
upper border of the Clavicle
posterior border of SCM

2 SCM

3 Clavicle

4 apex of the lung

5 Scalenius anterior muscle

5a access point for regional anaesthesia in muscle
note must be above the lung apex

6 Trapezius

7 site for anaesthesia for the BP
note above incision for access to subclavian vessels & adjacent structures

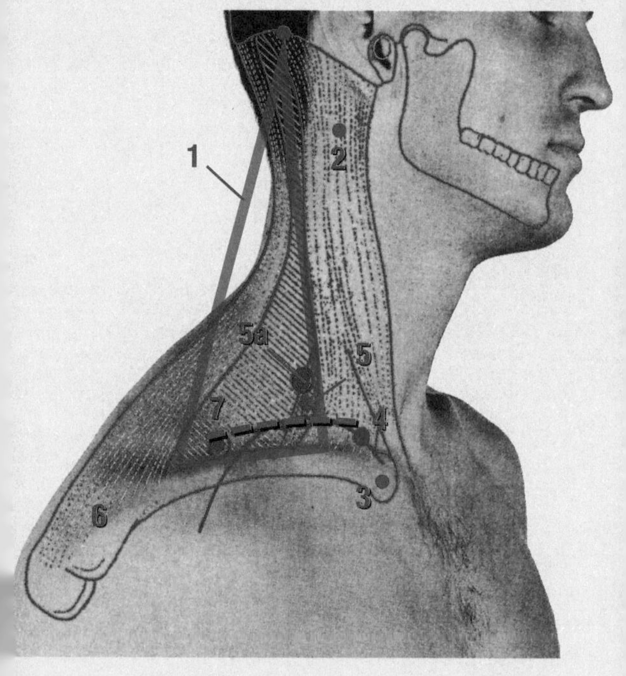
1
2
5a
5
7
4
3
6

Nose

anterior view

1 glabella

2 rhinion – b/n nasal bone and cartilage osseocartilagenous junction = root of nose

3 d = dorsum of nose t = tip defining points

4 supra alar crease

5 alar side wall

6 philtrum

inferior view

7 infratip nodule

8 columella

9 alar- facial junction (groove b/n nose and face)

10 nasal sill

11 facet = soft tissue triangle

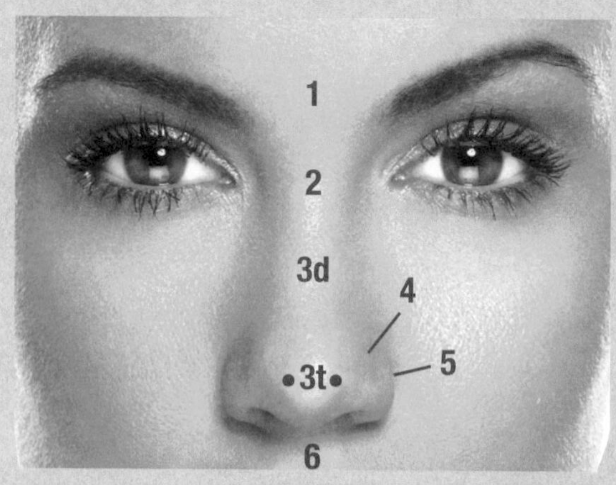
1
2
3d
4
5
•3t•
6

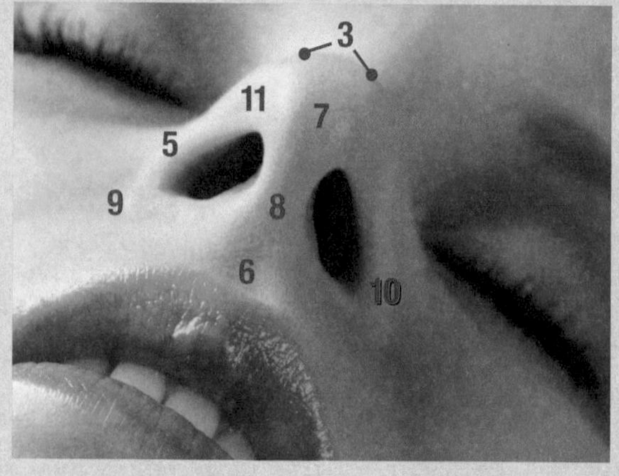
3
11
7
5
9
8
6
10

A

Nose – cartilages

B

Note the cartilages of the nose vary a great deal and determine the shape height and aesthetic and ethnic appearance of the nose.

C

D

anterior view

E

1 nasal bone

F

2 lateral cartilages - may be separated into superior and inferior cartilages

G

3 lesser alar cartilages

H

4 alar cartilages

I

5 fibrofatty tissue

J

6 philtrum

K

7 septal cartilage + fibrofatty tissue

8 nare

L

9 columella

M

N *inferio - medial view*

O

10 dorsum of the nose

P

11 dorsum of alar cartilages = tip defininig points

Q

12 alar facial folds = b/n alars & dermis

13 nare – deep inside the septal cartilage

R

14 alar cartilage lateral crus

S

15 alar cartilage medial crus

T

U

V

W

X

Y

Z

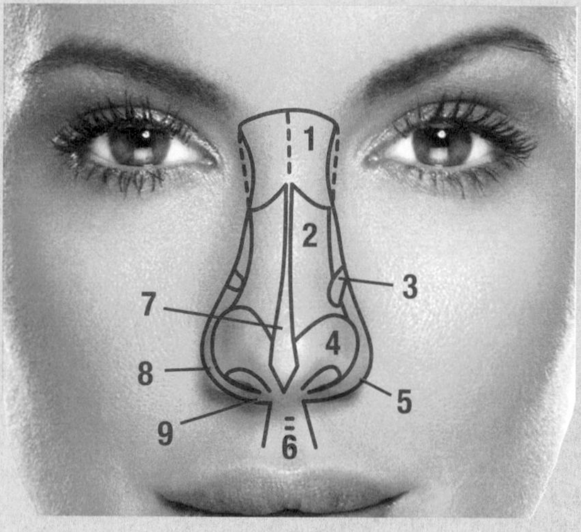

1
2
3
7
4
8
5
9
6

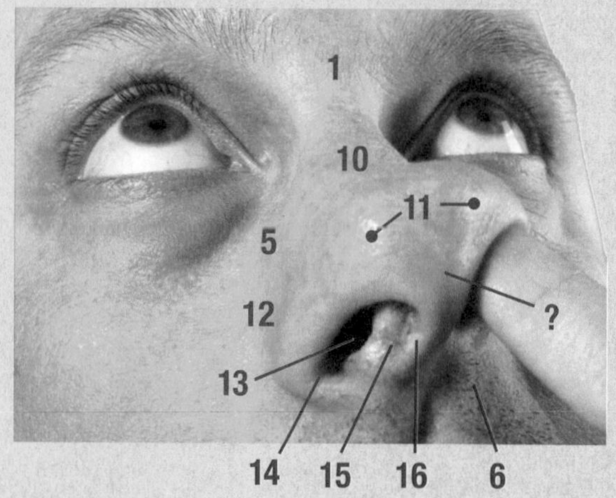
1
10
11
5
12
?
13
14
15
16
6

Nose – cartilages

Inferior view - mature nose

1 central nasal fibro fatty tissue – varies considerably

2 tip defining points on either side

3 septal cartilage

4 alar cartilage L = lateral crus , m = medial crus

5 alar facial fold

6 philtum

7 nasal spine – bone

8 nostril = naris (pl = nares)

9 nasal sill

10 fibrofatty tissue

Inferior view - immature nose

8 nostril – note absence of hair inside

10 fibrofatty tissue more extensive as cartilage incomplete nose is a lot softer and prone to collapse with pressure

11 columella – incomplete septal cartilage

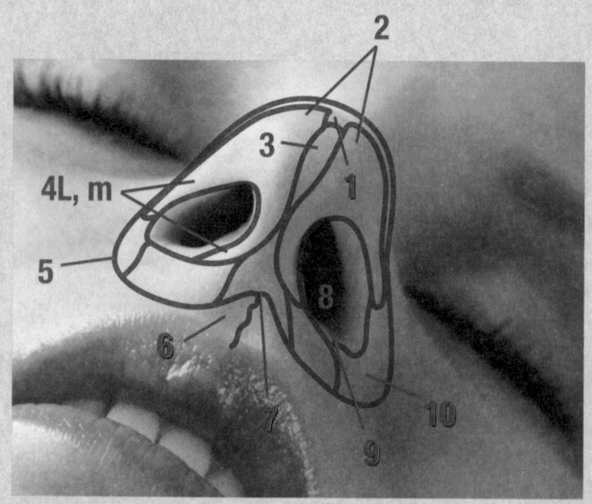
2
3
1
4L, m
5
8
6
7
10
9

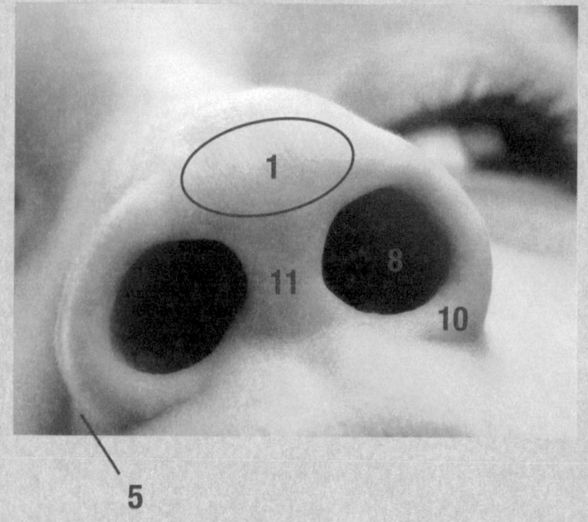
1
8
11
10
5

Nose

lateral view

1 glabella
2 nasion – angle b/n frontal & nasal bones
3 rhinion – osseocartilaginous junction
4 supra tip
5 tip defining points
6 philtrum
7 infratip nodule
8 columella
9 alar- facial junction (groove b/n nose and face)
10 nasal sill
11 nasolabial fold
12 alar sidewall

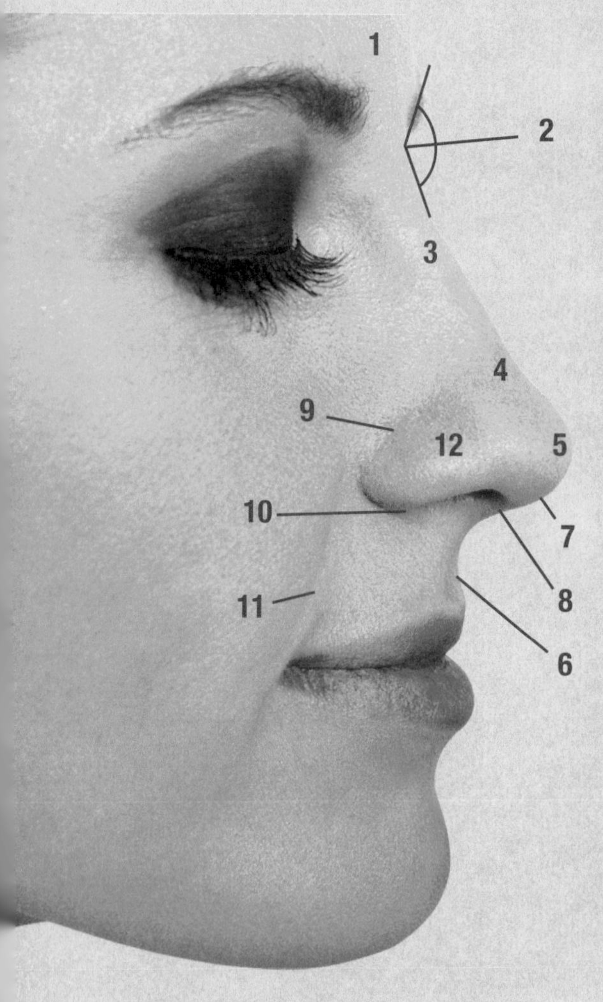
1
2
3
4
9
12
5
10
7
11
8
6

A B C D E F G H I J K L M **N** O P Q R S T U V W X Y Z

Nose – cartilages

Lateral view

There is considerable variation b/n the size and positioning of the cartilages, particularly the alar cartilages which are often repositioned in plastic surgery.

B/n the bone and cartilage there may be overlap and a ridge or bump may be present - which is also often altered in cosmetic surgery.

The cartilage may continue to grow into adulthood lengthening the nose, and growth of the fibrofatty tissue partic with retention of oily substances may widen and thicken the nose particularly in males.

1 nasal bone
2 lateral cartilage
3 septal cartilage
4 alar cartilage (major) 4m = minor alar cartilages
5 infra nasal tip
6 nasal opening
7 philtrum
8 nasolabial fold
9 fibro-fatty tissue
10 alar - facial junction

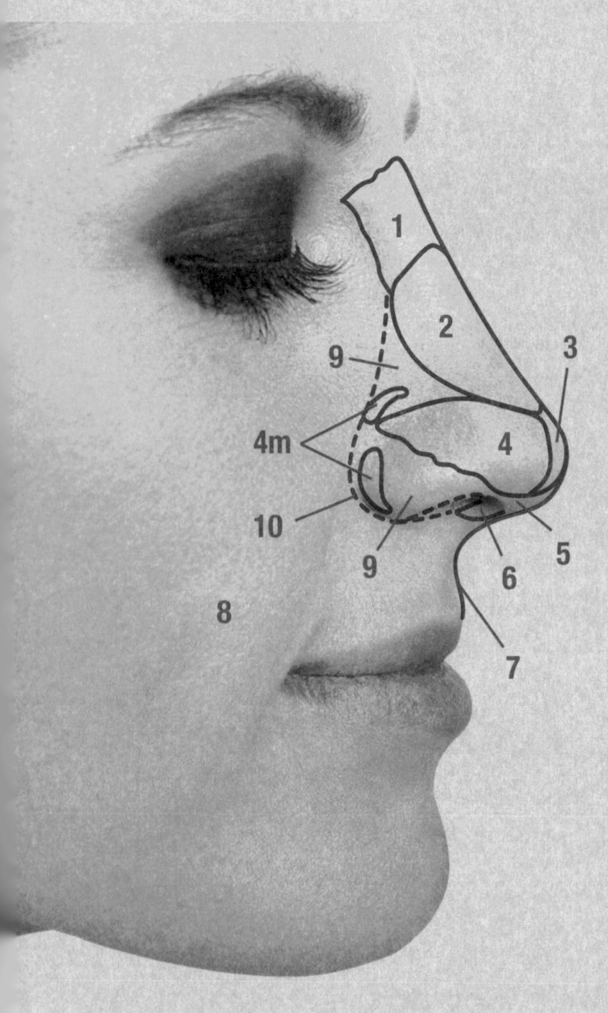
1
2
3
9
4m
4
10
9
5
6
8
7

Oesophagus, Phrenic N Vagus N

Anterior view

Demonstrating a projection of the oesophagus on the chest and relationship with the Phrenic & Vagus Ns.

1. Vagus N with recurrent laryngeal branches - note L lower than R wrapping around the aortic arch L & R
2. Phrenic N L & R
3. cardiac plexus
4. oesophagus

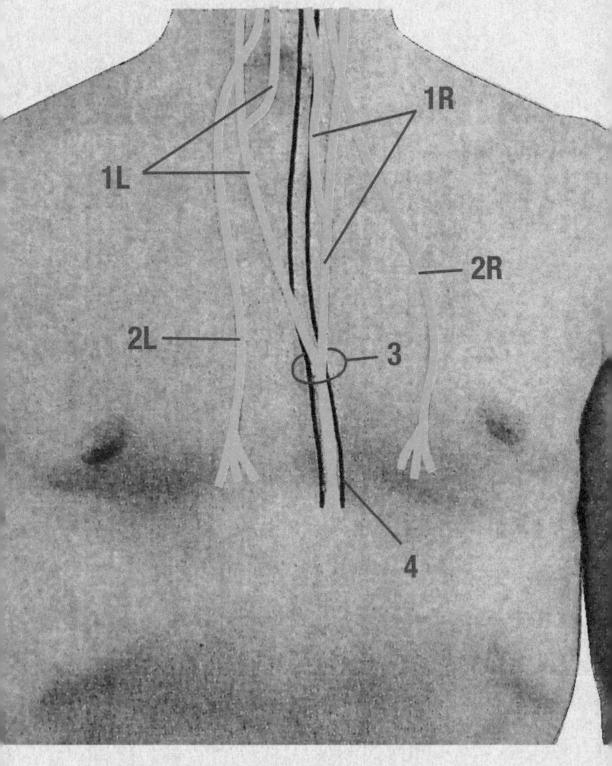
1R
1L
2R
2L
3
4

Penis
male genitalia

with foreskin – uncircumcised
w/o foreskin – circumcised

In the anatomical position the penis is described as erect however these images do not show this position - hence the shaft of the penis shown is the dorsal surface. Generally when examined the penis is not erect and hence this is the commoner position seen.

1 shaft of the penis - dorsal surface
2 foreskin - remnants remaining in the circumcised image
3 urethral opening
4 scrotum - sac containing the testes
5 glans penis - exposed in the circumcised penis

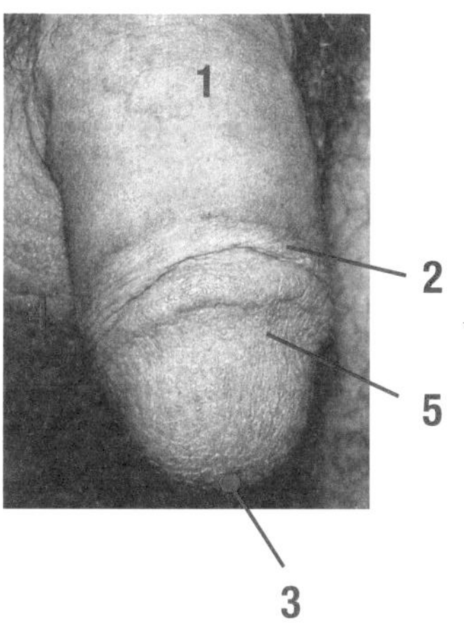

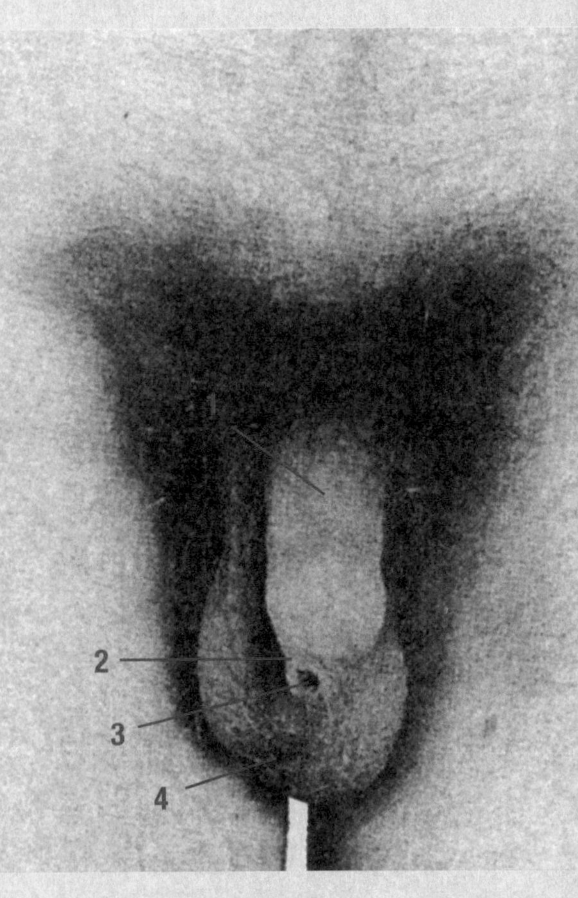
1
2
3
4

Pelvis / Perineum - Female
Bones

Inferior view -

showing the boney outlines of the female pelvis and perineum.

1 Clitoris

2 Labia Majora

3 uretheral opening

4 Labia Minora

5 vaginal opening

6 anal opening = Anus (with anal skin tag)

7 inferior pubic ramus

8 Acetabulum

9 ischeal tuberosity

10 sacral tuberous ligament

11 PIIS

12 Sacrum

13 Coccyx

14 Sacropinous ligament

15 Gluteus Maximus m

16 Hamstring muscles

17 Adductor Magnus m

18 Gracilis m

19 Adductor Longus m

20 perineal body

A B C D E F G H I J K L M N O **P** Q R S T U V W X Y Z

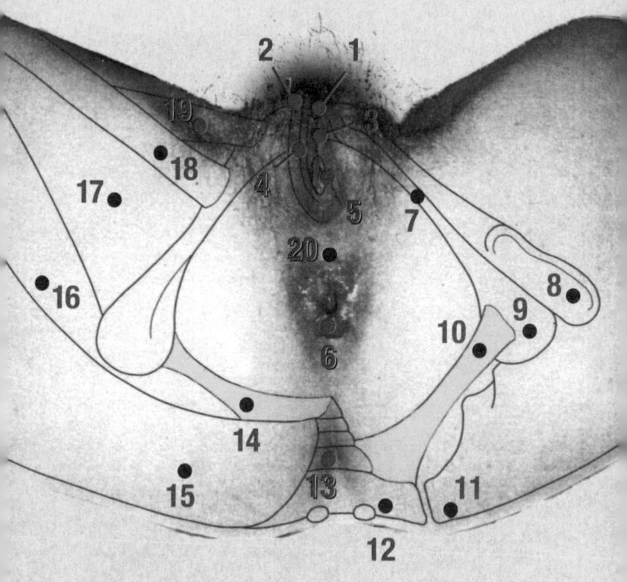
2
1
19
3
18
4
17
5
7
20
8
16
9
10
6
14
13
11
15
12

A B C D E F G H I J K L M N O **P** Q R S T U V W X Y Z

Pelvis / Perineum - Female Muscles

Inferior view -
showing the muscles of the female perineum.

1 Ischiocavernous m
2 Transverse perinei superficialis m
3 Levator Ani m
4 Gluteus maximus m
5 External anal sphincter
6 Bulbospongiosus m
7 perineal body

Male Dermatomes

The inferior surface of the Perineum is innervated by L2-S5.

The skin surrounding the anus and vagina/scrotal sac is innervated by S4/5.

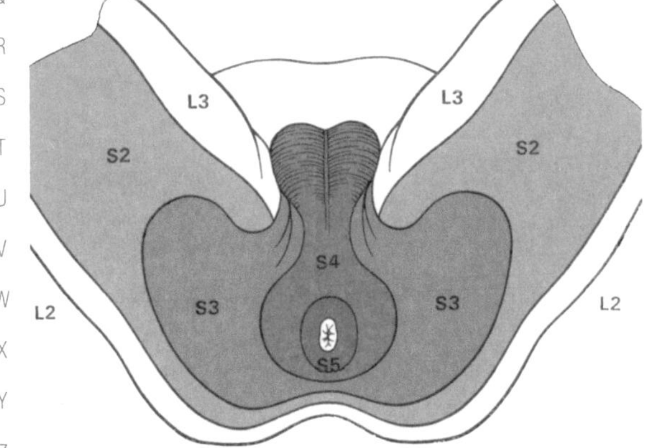

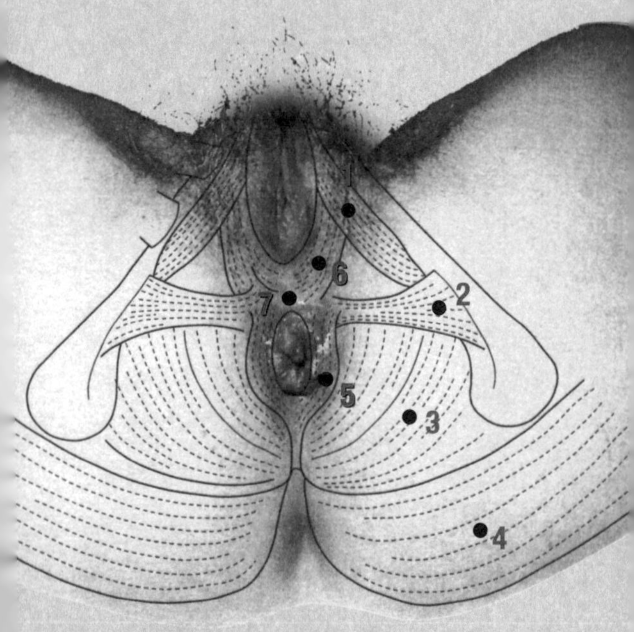
1
2
3
4
5
6
7

A B C D E F G H I J K L M N O **P** Q R S T U V W X Y Z

Popliteal Fossa

BVs & Ns

The popliteal fossa lies at the back of the knee and is equivalent to the cubital fossa in the arm. Clinically it is an important site, often the site of aneurysms and DVT. "Baker's cyst"

1 Adductor hiatus
2 Popliteal artery & vein
3 Biceps femoris m
4 Tibial N
5 Common Peroneal N
6 Tibial artery a = anterior p = posterior
7 Peroneal artery

Muscles & Bones

8 Gastrocnemius
L = lateral head
m = medial head
9 Semitendinous m
10 Semimembranous m
11 Gracilis m
12 Sartorius m

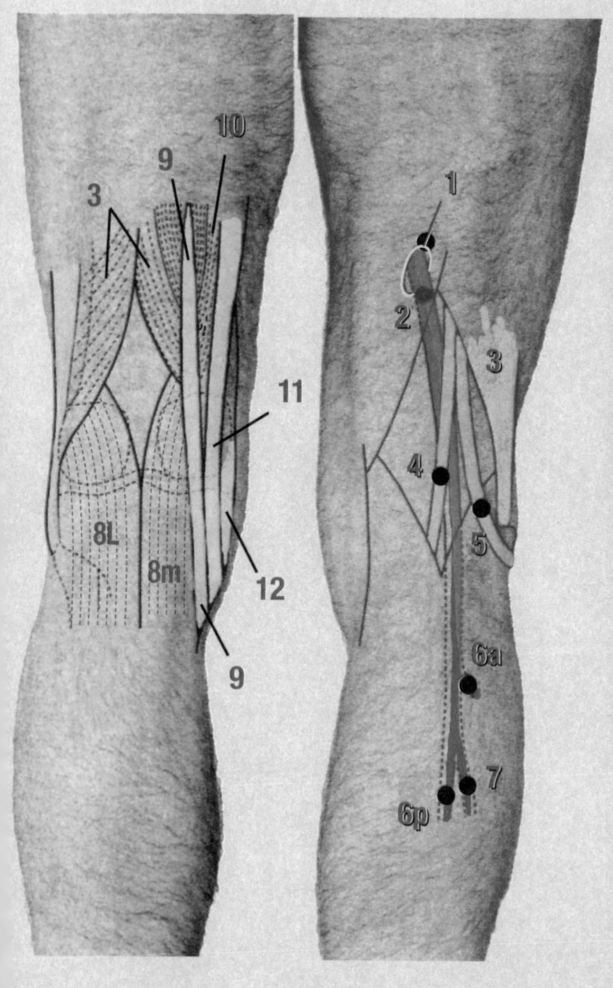
10
9
3
11
8L
8m
12
9
1
2
3
4
5
6a
7
6p

Sciatic Nerve

Posterior

Surface projection of the Sciatic N pathway - showing vulnerable sites and site for injection - upper outer quadrant of the buttock.

N emerges midway b/n PSIS (1) and the ischeal tuberosity (2) moves posteriorly near the acetabulum (hence may be damaged in hip surgery) and may split into the lateral and medial branches (medial & lateral popliteal Ns respectively) in the gluteal region at the level of the Greater trochanter (3) or remain as one N until entering the lower limb.

It is under the cover of the Gluteus Maximus but is exposed in the upper thigh, before going under Biceps Femoris.

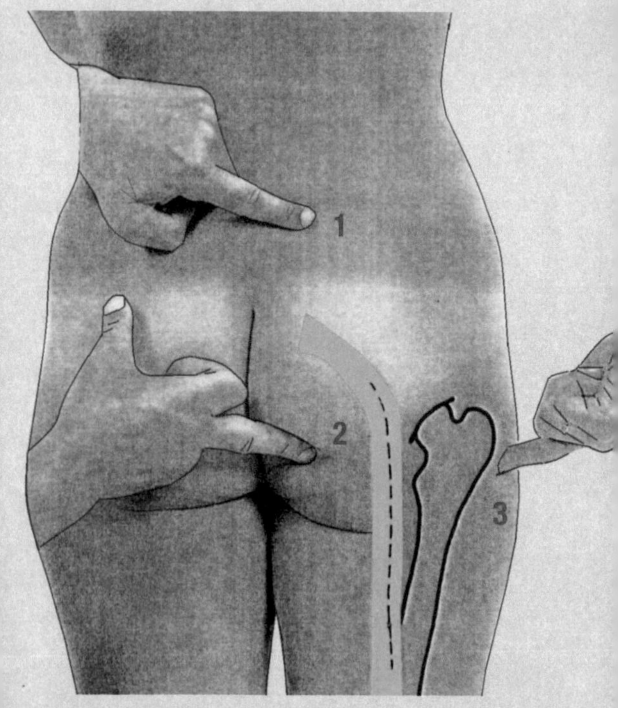
1
2
3

Shoulder – Upper arm

Bones

Anterior view

1 sternoclavicular joint
2 Clavicle
3 1st rib
4 costoclavicular ligament
5 coracoclavicular ligaments
6 Acromion
7 7g = greater tuberosity 7L = lesser tuberosity (of the Humerus)
8 bicipital groove
9 coracoid process
10 glenohumeral joint / shoulder joint
11 Humerus

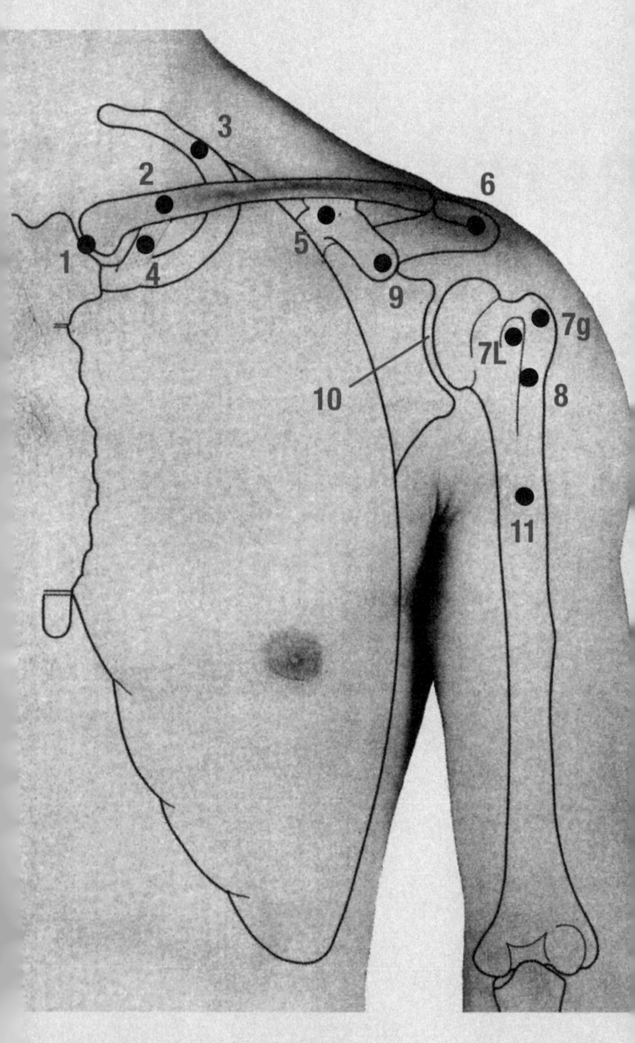
3
2
6
1
5
4
9
7g
7L
10
8
11

A
Shoulder – Upper arm
B
BVs & Ns
C
Anterior views
D
E
1 Brachial Plexus trunks (separated out for clarity)
F
2 common carotid artery
3 subclavian vein and site of access for vessel
G
4 Clavicle
H
5 Pectoralis minor m
I
6 Median N
J
7 radial & ulnar arteries (terminal branches of the Brachial art)
K
8 subclavian artery - name changes with position
L
i = subclavian
M
ii = axillary
iii = brachial arteries
N
O
P
Q
R
S
T
U
V
W
X
Y
Z

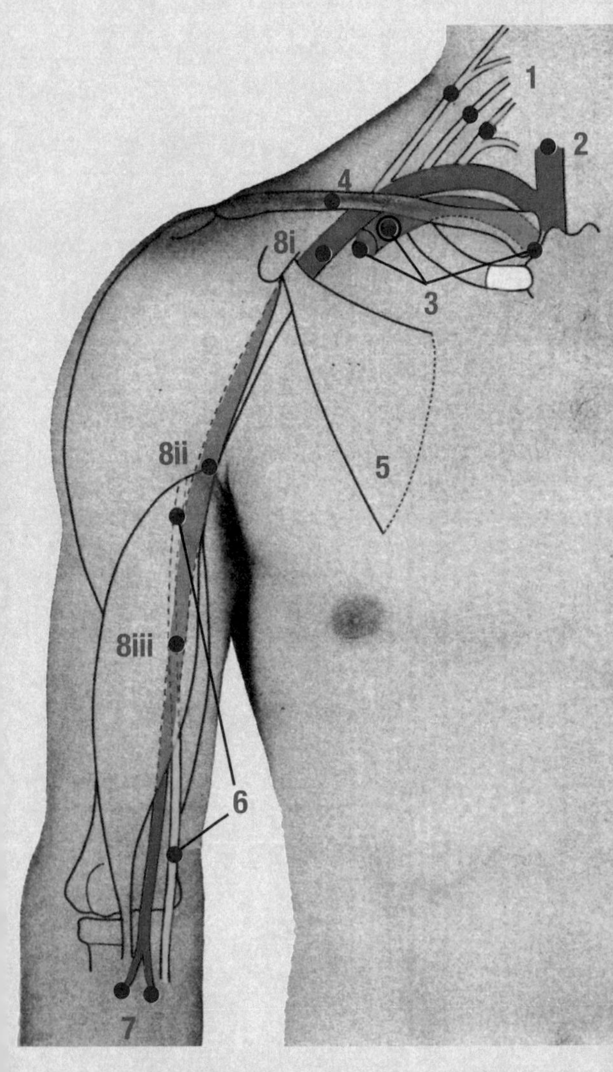
1
2
4
8i
3
5
8ii
8iii
6
7

A B C D E F G H I J K L M N O P Q R **S** T U V W X Y Z

Shoulder – Upper arm muscles

Anterior

1 Clavicle
2 Acromion
3 Humerus
4 Pectoralis major
   c = clavicular head
   s = sternocostal head
5 Deltoid a = anterior L = lateral p = posterior fibres
6 Scapula s = spine of

Superior

view of Deltoid muscle capping the shoulder.

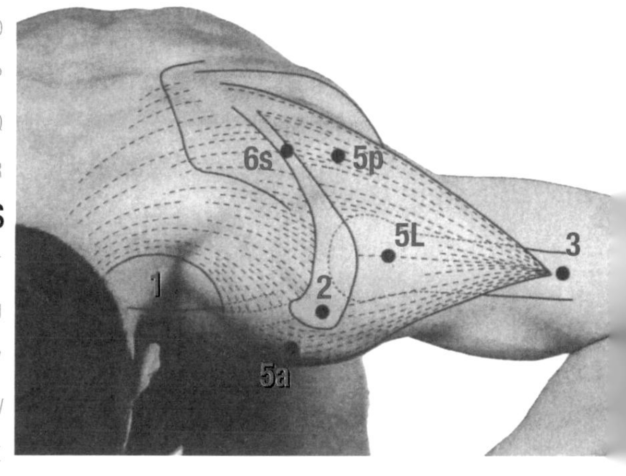

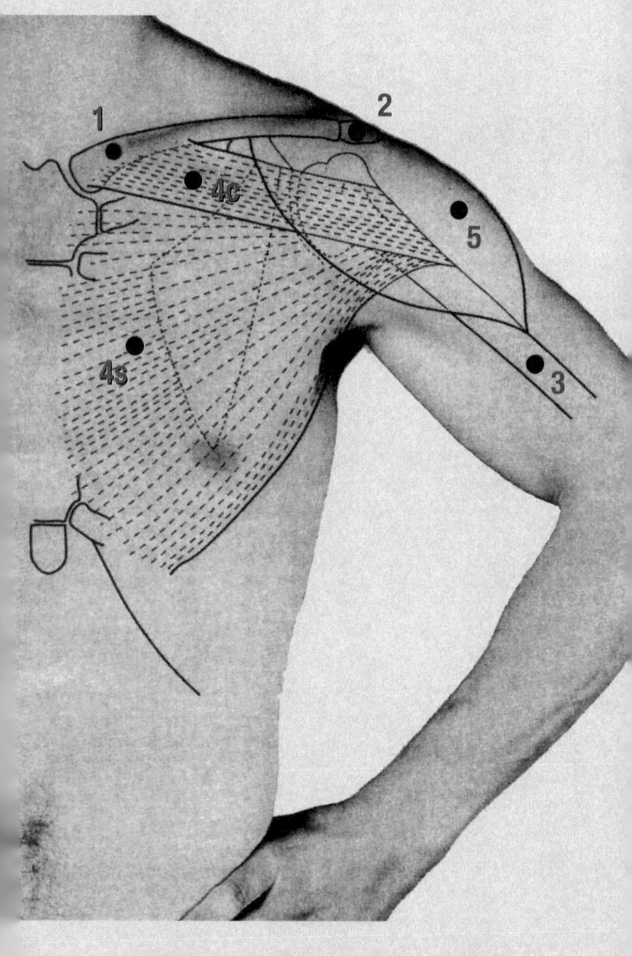
1
2
4c
5
4s
3

A B C D E F G H I J K L M N O P Q R **S** T U V W X Y Z

Shoulder – Upper arm muscles - deep

Posterior

1 Supraspinatus m
2 Acromion
3 Humerus
4 Teres minor m
5 Deltoid outline –
muscles shown are deep to this muscle
6 Scapula m = medial edge (shoulder blade)
s = spine of
7 Infraspinatus m
8 Triceps m
i = long head
ii = medial head
iii = lateral head
9 radial N
10 axillary N
11 Teres major
12 Anconeus m

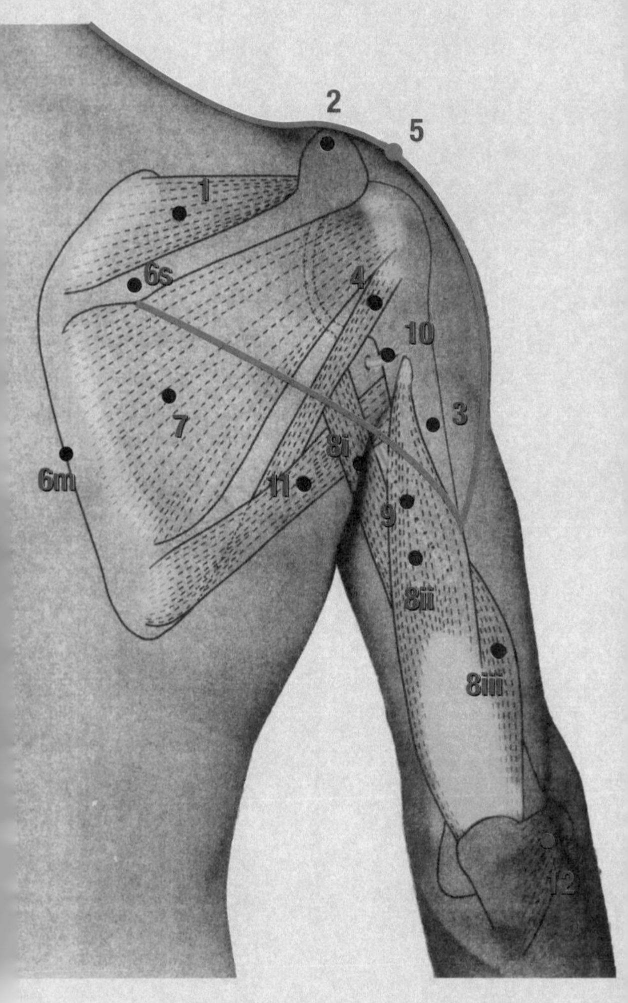
2
5
1
6s
4
10
7
3
6m
8i
11
9
8ii
8iii
12

A B C D E F G H I J K L M N O P Q R **S** T U V W X Y Z

Shoulder – Upper arm muscles – superficial

Posterior

1 Trapezius m

2 Acromion

3 Humerus

4 Latissimus Dorsi m

5 Deltoid m

6 Scapula m = medial edge (shoulder blade)
s = spine of
i = superior angle
ii = medial angle
iii = inferior angle

7 glenoid fossa

8 Levator Scapulae m

9 Supraspinatus m

10 i = Teres minor
ii = Teres major muscle

11 Infraspinatus m

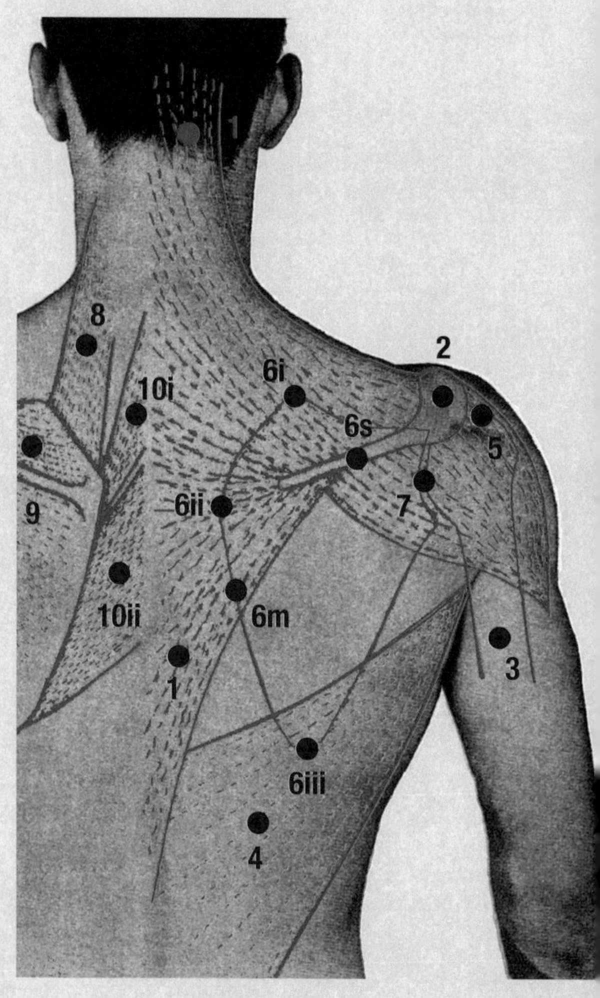
1
8
2
6i
10i
6s
5
7
6ii
9
10ii
6m
3
1
6iii
4

A

Sinuses

B

Anterior view

C

Surface projection of the sinuses of the Head onto the face.

D Dotted lines indicate how extensive the sinuses may be - they may extend to the teeth and across the forehead.

E

1 frontal sinus
2 ethmoid sinus
3 air cells b/n orbits
4 maxillary sinus
5 upper jaw and teeth

F G H I J K L M N O P Q R **S** T U V W X Y Z

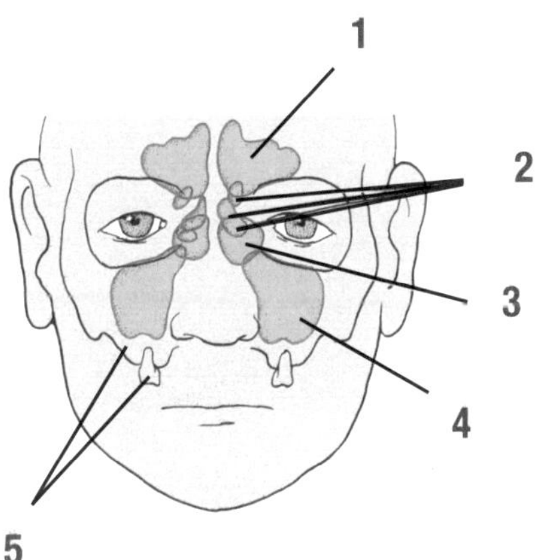

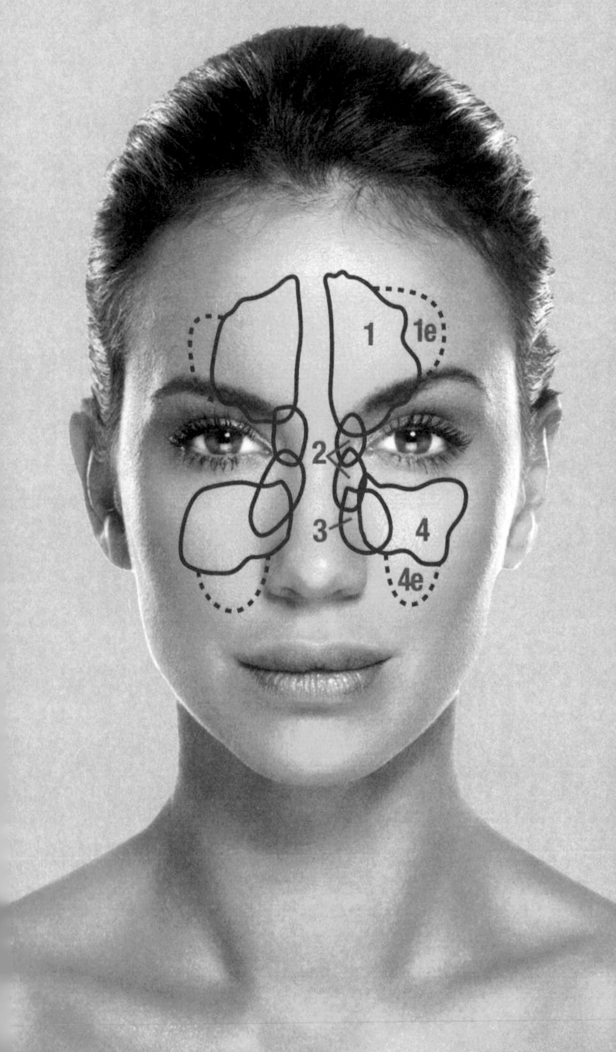
1
1e
2
3
4
4e

Spleen

Anterior view

Surface projection of the spleen showing its relation to the pancreas

Lateral view

Surface projection showing its relation to the ribs

The spleen occupies the LUQ, pressed up against the diaphragm. It is generally covered by ribs 9-11 but may extend deep into the abdominal space in disease, particularly parasitic diseases. It is a soggy bag of blood with a fragile capsule so that if exposed due to splenomegaly, it may be easily injured and bleed into the abdominal cavity.

1 spleen
   e = enlarged (splenomegaly)
   p = enlarged due to parasites extending into the abdominal cavity
2 transpyloric plane = L1
3 L kidney
4 L4
5 L5
6 pancreas - head inserted into the 2nd part of the duodenum
7 R adrenal gland
8 xiphisternum
9 rib 9
10 rib 10
11 rib 11

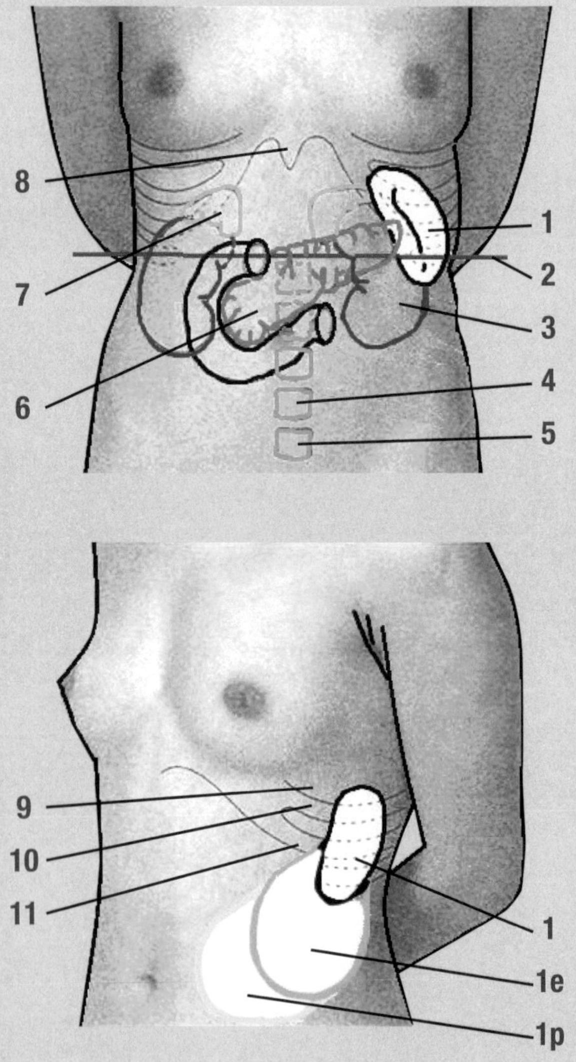
8
1
7
2
3
6
4
5
9
10
11
1
1e
1p

Stomach

unseen 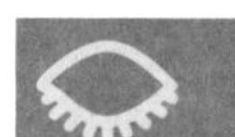

Anterior

Surface projection of the stomach showing changes in the position from supine to upright. May fall as much as 6cm.

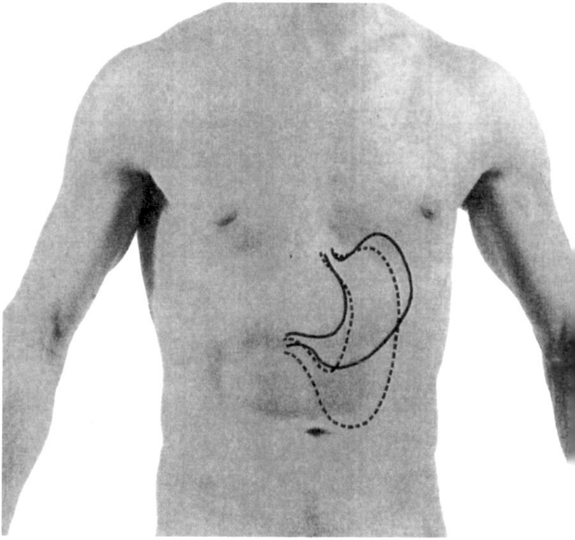

A B C D E F G H I J K L M N O P Q R **S** T U V W X Y Z

Stomach - position changes

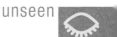

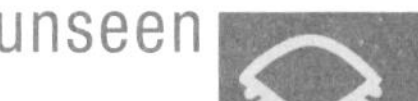

Anterior

The Stomach is a highly mobile organ. It can contain up to 2 litres of food. The body is not fixed – but the oesophageal and pyloric regions are. The muscle layers of the stomach contract and force the food towards the pyloris whatever its shape making it very functionally very adaptable. Note despite many restrictive surgeries (as in gastric banding) the stomach manages to continue to function well.

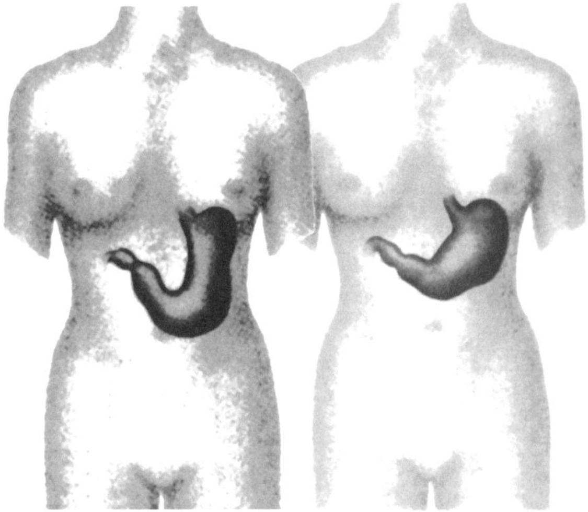

normal

active

A B C D E F G H I J K L M N O P Q R **S** T U V W X Y Z

Here are examples of 4 different states of a normal stomach.

1 normal
2 actively digesting
3 stretched
4 pregnant*

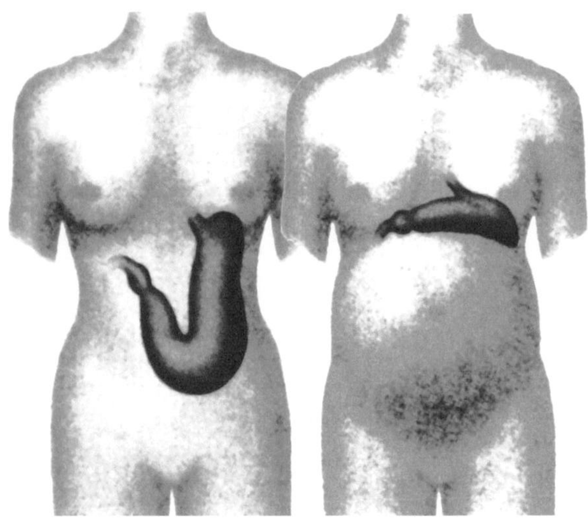

stretched pregnant

*It is easy to see why dyspepsia and indigestion is common in pregnancy and obesity.

Temporomandibular joint

Lateral view

open / shut

The TMJ is the only synovial joint in the head and is highly unstable, although it moves with chewing - in normal chewing there is no significant pressure on this joint

Grinding of teeth at night – Inflammation of the temporal artery may effect this joint and cause severe headaches.

1 Zygomatic arch - cheek bone

2 TML- moves when opening or closing the jaw palpate in front of the tragus - articulating surface with the condyle of the Mandible

3 EAM = external auditory meatus

4 mastoid process

5 spinous process

6 Mandible
a = angle
c = coronoid process of
r = ramus

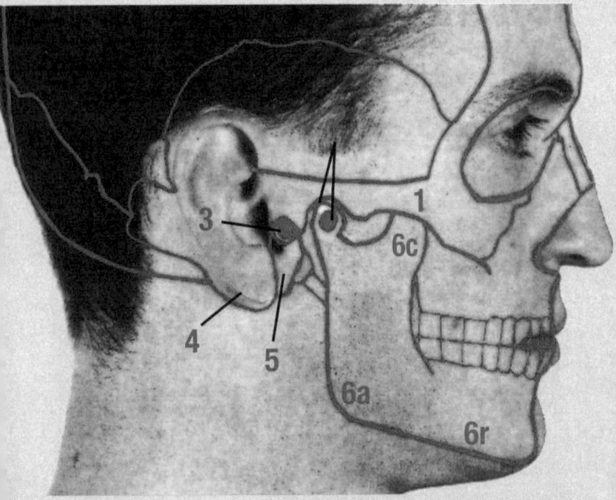

1
3
6c
4
5
6a
6r
1 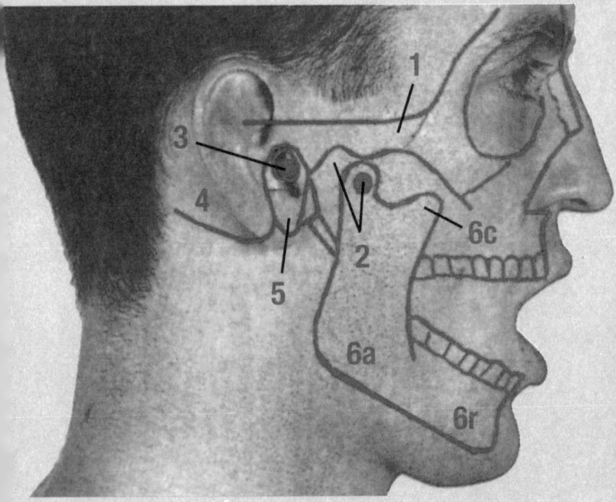
3
4
6c
2
5
6a
6r

Testis

Anterio-lateral

view of the Scrotum - penis moved aside.

The testes are contained in the scrotal sac. They can be palpated along with the spermatic cord exiting the abdomen/pelvis via the external inguinal ring

L testis generally lies lower than the R as it desends first

– comma – shaped 3X4-5 cm

May contract on examination particularly in adolescent boys due to the cremaster muscle (inserted in the mesentery of the testis) - cremasteric reflex

1 external inguinal ring
2 spermatic cord
3 vas deferens = ductus deferens contained w/in the cord
4 epididymis - superior pole
5 testis
6 inguinal ligament

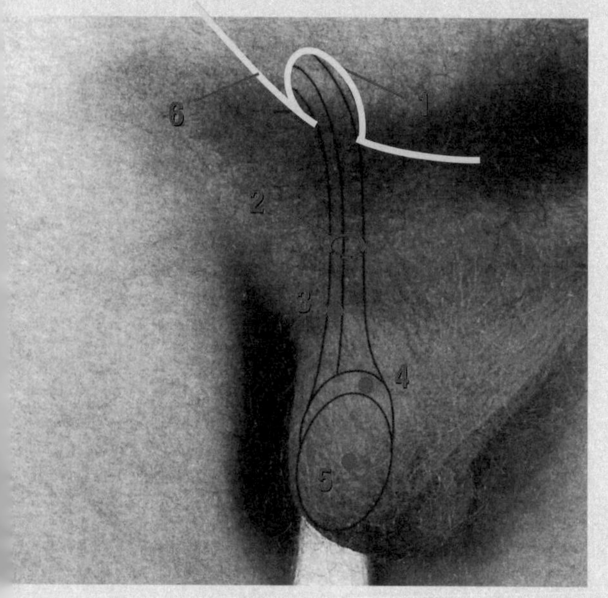
1
2
3
4
5
6

Thigh
Muscle

Anterior view

1 ASIS
2 Obturator Externus m
3 hip joint
4 Abductor Brevis m
5 Abductor Magnus m
6 Abductor hiatus
7 Patella t = tendon
8 Tibia
9 Vasti muscles all inserting into the Patella
i = intermedius
l = lateralis
m = medialis
10 Abductor Longus m
deep to the Abductors are the smaller hip rotating muscles
11 Pectineus m
12 Sartorius m
13 Tensor fascia lata m
14 Gracilis m
15 pelvic brim

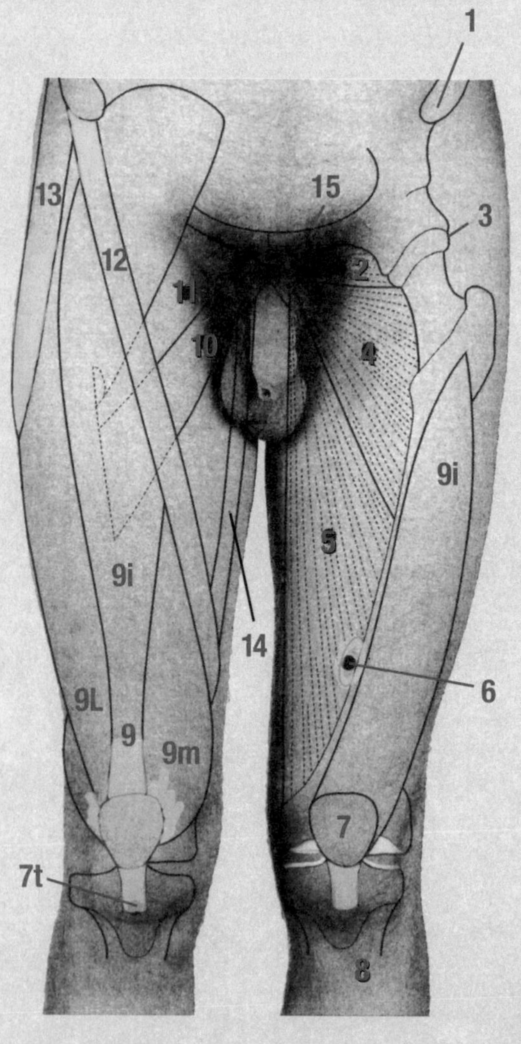
1
13
15
3
12
2
11
10
4
9i
9i
5
14
6
9L
9
9m
7
7t
8

A
Thumb – Anatomical snuff box

B
Bones

C 1 Ph = Phalanges d = distal, p = proximal
D 2 MC – 1st metacarpal
E 3 Trapezium
F 4 Scaphoid
5 Radius s = styloid process, t = dorsal tubercle
G
H
Tendons

I
6 extensor pollicus longus
J 7 extensor carpi radialis longus
K 8 extensor carpi brevis
L 9 abductor pollicus longus
M 10 extensor pollicus brevis

N
O
BVs and Ns

P 11 cephalic vein
12 radial N
Q 13 radial artery

R
S
T
U
V
W
X
Y
Z

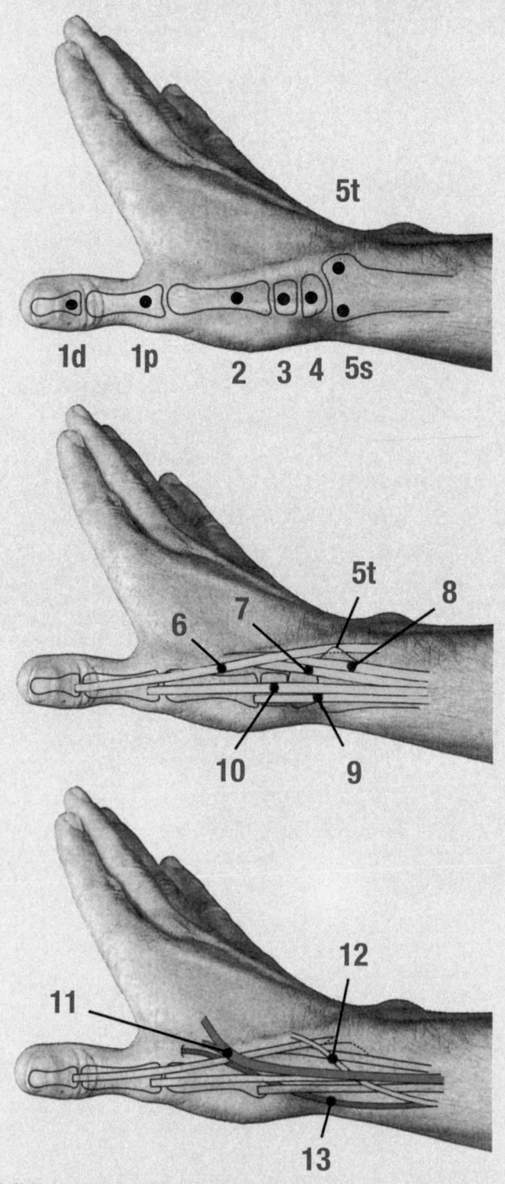
5t
1d
1p
2
3
4
5s
5t
8
7
6
10
9
12
11
13

A
B
C
D
E
F
G
H
I
J
K
L
M
N
O
P
Q
R
S
T
U
V
W
X
Y
Z

Thymus

Anterior -

showing relationship to Oesophagus & anterior chest.

Borders - Manubrium - 4th CC, immediately behind Manubriosternum anterior to the heart - may vary in size and position - larger in children.

1 Oesophagus

2 Thymus – R & L

3 Manbubriosternum

Thyroid

Anterior -

showing relationship to Hyoid bone and cervical cartilages.

Parathyroid glands lie behind the thyroid but may be found in the thorax - near the thymus.

4 Hyoid bone - body and greater horn

5 Thyroid cartilage = Adam's apple

5-6 Cricothyroid membrane

6 Cricoid cartilage

7 1st tracheal ring

8 isthmus of the thyroid gland
5L lobe of thyroid (R & L lobes) growth in the lobes produces obvious protrusion - goitre in the neck

9 medial border of SCM

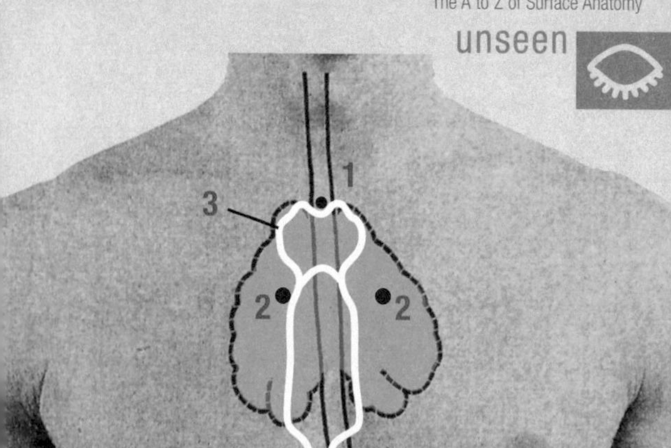

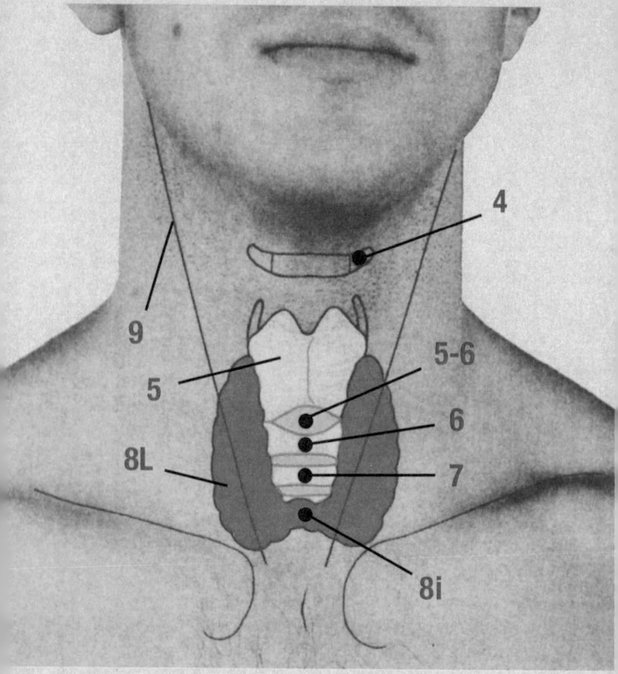

4
9
5-6
5
6
8L
7
8i

Tongue

Protruding tongue – open mouth anterolateral anterior

The tongue is protruded in order to see the uvula and should poke straight out if there is a lesion of the CN XII = Hypoglossal N it will deviate to the side of the lesion.

If there is a lesion of the pharyngeal br of the Vagus N (CN X) the uvula will appear uneven also with deviation to the side of the lesion.

The surface of a healthy tongue appears even, fleshy and pink – coating may indicate infection particularly of candidiasis, it is also a common site of tumours and should be examined thoroughly on

1 median lingual sulcus
2 apex
3 body of the tongue
4 palatine tonsil
5 lingual tonsil
6 circumvallate papillae - at the sulcus terminalis - end of the tongue
7 uvula

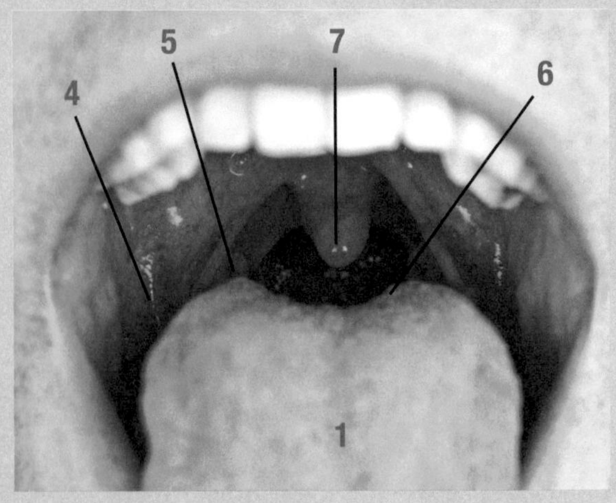
5
7
6
4
1

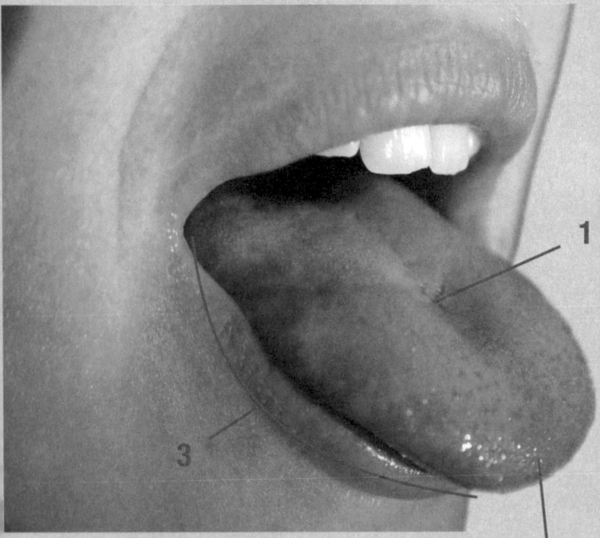

1
3
2

Tongue

Elevated tongue

The tongue is a large very mobile skeletal muscle innervated by the Hypoglossal N.

Piercings may be seen through the median lingual sulcus, which splits the tongue muscle in 2 with symmetrical muscles on either side.

Splitting allows for increased mobility but interferes with speech.

1 naso-labial fold
2 radial art more medial than the ...
3 lingual N
4 tongue
a = apex b = body r = root of the tongue
5 median lingual sulcus
6 frenulum
7 sublingual salivary gland o = opening

A B C D E F G H I J K L M N O P Q R S **T** U V W X Y Z

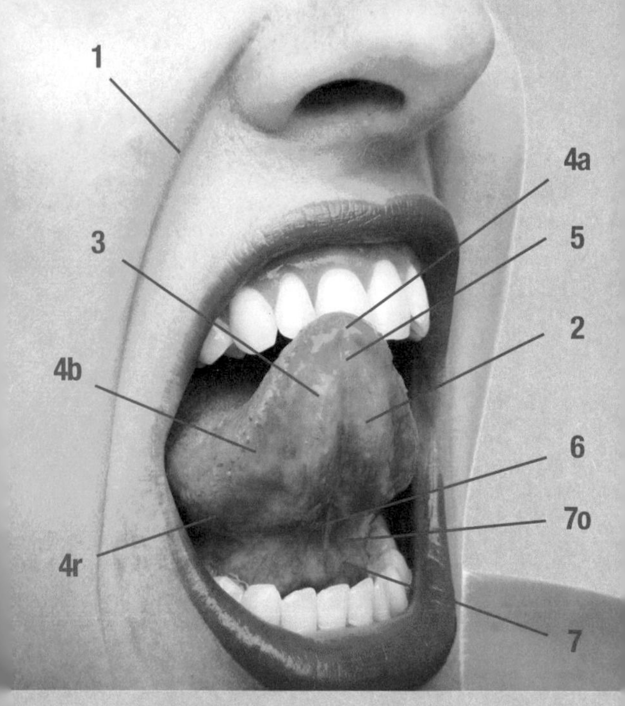
1
4a
3
5
2
4b
6
7o
4r
7

Trachea

Lateral view

of trachea showing the more prominent male cricoid cartilage = Adam's apple.

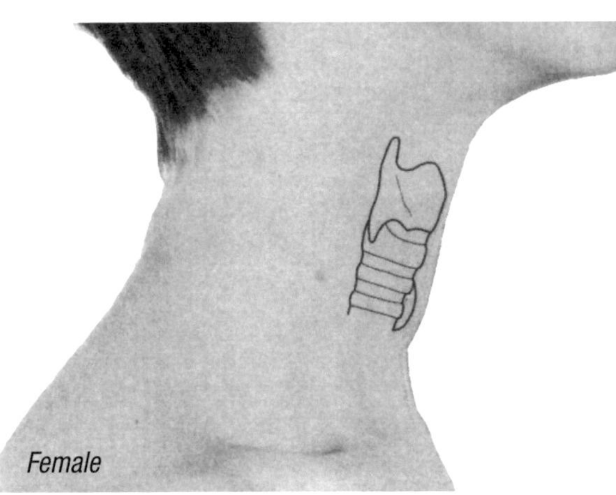

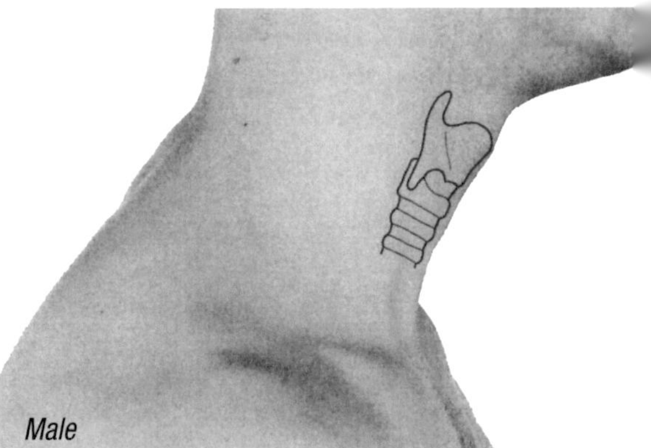

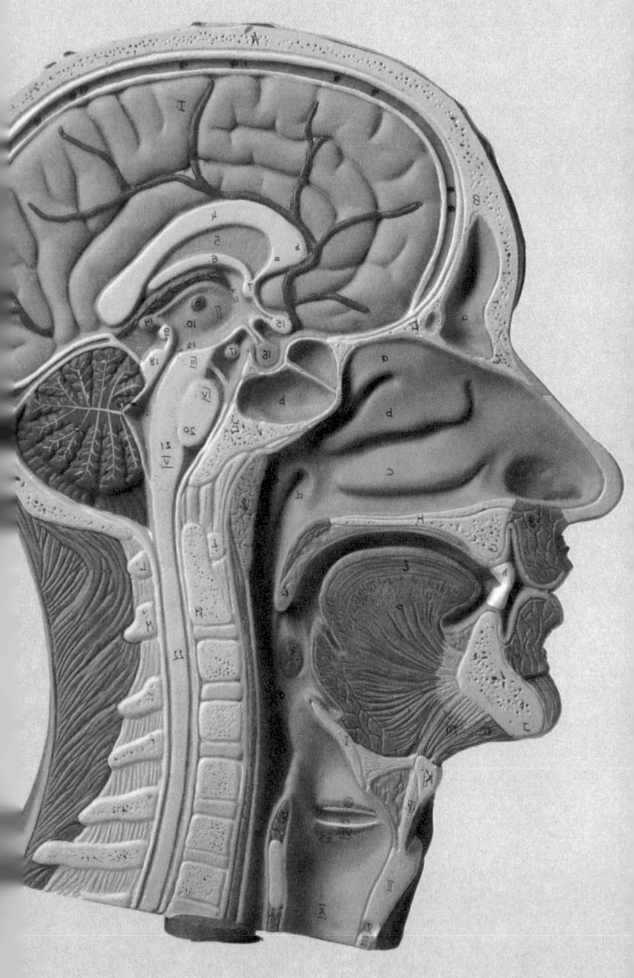

A B C D E F G H I J K L M N O P Q R S T **U** V W X Y Z

Uterus
Ovaries
Bladder

Anterior view

of female internal genitalia and relationship with bladder.

1 ovary
2 fallopian tube = ovarian tube
3 bladder – e = empty / resting
f = full – well above the pelvic brim completely covering the uterus*
4 uterus
5 urethra

Note the full bladder rising above the pelvic brim and covering the uterus – pushes the other abdominal organs up into the abdomen and permits an unobstructed view (ultrasound) of the uterine contents

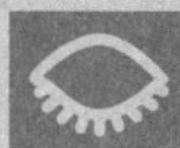

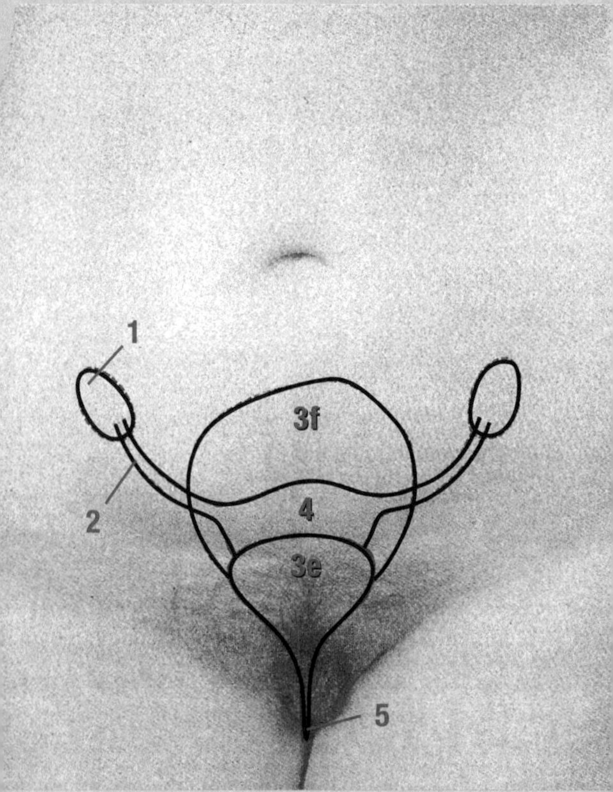

1
3f
2
4
3e
5

Forearm / Wrist Tendons

Anterior

Arteries large and medium have a similar structure.

1 radial styloid
2 flexor carpi radialis
3 palmaris longus
4 flexor carpi ulnaris
5 palmaris brevis

A B C D E F G H I J K L M N O P Q R S T U V **W** X Y Z

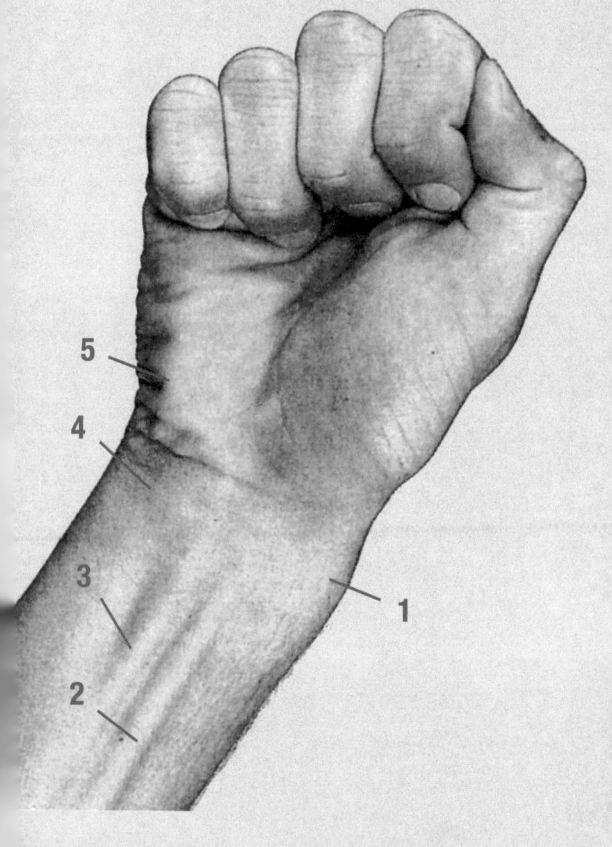
5
4
3
2
1